The Chic Closet

*Inspired ideas to develop
your personal style,
fall in love with your
wardrobe, and bring back the
joy of dressing yourself*

FIONA FERRIS

Copyright © 2020 Fiona Ferris
www.howtobechic.com
All rights reserved.

ISBN: 9798690075149

Other books by Fiona Ferris

Thirty Chic Days: *Practical inspiration for a beautiful life*

Thirty More Chic Days: *Creating an inspired mindset for a magical life*

Thirty Slim Days: *Create your slender and healthy life in a fun and enjoyable way*

Financially Chic: *Live a luxurious life on a budget, learn to love managing money, and grow your wealth*

How to be Chic in the Winter: *Living slim, happy and stylish during the cold season*

A Chic and Simple Christmas: *Celebrate the holiday season with ease and grace*

The Original 30 Chic Days Blog Series: *Be inspired by the online series that started it all*

30 Chic Days at Home: *Self-care tips for when you have to stay at home, or any other time when life is challenging*

The Chic Author: *Create your dream career and lifestyle, writing and self-publishing non-fiction books*

Treinta Días Chic: *Inspiración practica para una vida hermosa (Spanish Edition)*

FIONA FERRIS

Contents

Introduction 1

Chapter 1. *Invite your muse to play* 5

Chapter 2. *Fall in love with your current wardrobe* 11

Chapter 3. *Develop your style with a personal brand* 18

Chapter 4. *Cultivating the 'expensive' look* 26

Chapter 5. *Inject excitement with a capsule* du mois 33

Chapter 6. *Claiming 'sexiness' as a state of mind* 39

Chapter 7. *Creating your own fashion uniform* . 43

Chapter 8. *Decluttering your closet with inspiration* 49

Chapter 9. *The spiritual aspect to looking after your clothes* 55

Chapter 10. The two-colour rule 60

Chapter 11. Inspiring yourself to slim with your wardrobe..65

Chapter 12. Fashion versus style a la *Coco Chanel 71*

Chapter 13. How to be a frugal fashionista.........76

Chapter 14. Creating the perfect wardrobe for you 82

Chapter 15. Be inspired by men 90

Chapter 16. The chic lingerie drawer 96

Chapter 17. Lay out your clothes 101

21 top tips for a chic closet 106

A note from the author 116

About the author 119

Introduction

Welcome to *The Chic Closet*, a petite little book intended as a zippy read to inspire stylish action. In these pages I hope to rekindle your enthusiasm for dreaming up your most authentic and idealistic self; to dress yourself in a way that makes you zing with happiness; and build supreme confidence that you can look your very best, by dressing in a way that suits the task, while at the same time showcasing your own point of view.

And of course, not having to spend hours putting things together nor spending thousands on new clothes. For me, I like things to be easy, quick, and fun. If something takes too long, I don't want the bother, and this book follows the same spirit.

The Chic Closet is a mix of new material, and chapters inspired by favourite posts from my blog *How to be Chic*. I would just like to warn you straight up that this book about clothing and style *has no pictures*. The reason for this is that when I read a book with words only, it lets me concoct visuals in my mind. I often find that pictures put a very narrow vision in front of me, and I cannot translate the narrative to fit into my own life, style, or body shape. The way that my mind – and my writing – works, is that the inspiration I dream up and the words I use, inspires the mind to start thinking up ideas and new things to try.

Also, pictures date, even if you choose what you consider to be classic style to illustrate your point. I propose that the most fruitful way to approach dressing yourself is to use inspired ideas which can be applied over and over to *your* wardrobe, regardless of the current fashions. I have style books from decades past that I adore, however I wish they didn't have the eighties fashions to distract me. I have often thought that if the same book were brought out on Kindle with text only, that the reader could have a completely different experience and likely receive more value from the principles offered.

My most sincere wish with this book is that you jump up, half-way through a chapter and go to your wardrobe to put a new look together that you haven't tried before, or start re-organizing on a whim and loving the results. If you are not at home when this happens you will have to make do with some notes, or simply start visualizing what it is that has popped into your mind.

I feel confident that these impulsive actions will happen to you because they have happened to me too (and it is quite fun). As I wrote this book, I became more and more enthused about my own personal style. It is so gratifying to get the fun and excitement back into something that gave you immense pleasure at various stages of your life, but that perhaps you have gone a bit flat on at the moment. I am sure at some time in the past, maybe the very distant past, you were excited about dressing yourself. I can remember the thrill of looking at new season items as a teen and in my early twenties, and working out which ones I could afford for my wardrobe, or channelling the essence of something if it was outside of my budget.

Over the years my enthusiasm for style has increased and it has also been less. When it is more, the world seems brighter. And it is not just because I have been shopping either. When I think positively about my own personal style, it makes the clothes I already own seem more appealing.

In *The Chic Closet*, I am thrilled to share my favourite ways to inject excitement into the art of dressing. I don't consider myself a fashionista, even if it's fun to see the latest trends come out; rather, I am someone who desires to develop their own personal style over time. Because it is an evolving thing; we may change as the years go by, but we always carry our truth forward with us.

What I like about being on top of things with my wardrobe too, is that I can get ready quickly and easily in the morning – *with no angst* – and then forget about what I am wearing for the rest of the day because I am happy with my outfit. This book is all about style with comfort, elegance with thrift, appropriateness with playfulness and femininity with practicality.

I am so excited to take this creative style journey with you – thank you for joining me!

With all my best,

Fiona

Chapter 1.
Invite your muse to play

Let's start at the beginning and think about the possibilities a clean slate would afford us. Imagine if we could go back to a completely empty closet and have the ability to build our look from the ground up. Most of us will never get the chance to do this (or even want to), but it's a fun thing to think about and can give surprising insights.

One of my long-time favourite authors Brian Tracy calls this 'zero-based thinking'. He applies it to business, but you can equally apply to any part of your life, including your closet. Brian says to ask yourself, "Is there anything I'm doing today, that knowing what I now know, I wouldn't get into again if I had to do it over?"

So, with your wardrobe, you could ask yourself, "If I had to rebuy all of these clothes again, would I choose them?" Or "If I could dress in any way I liked, would I choose these styles?"

When I ponder questions like this, my Paris girl comes to mind. Not a Paris girl in real life, but the me I might be if I lived in a chic little apartment in the centre of Paris, with a view of the Eiffel Tower from my tiny iron balcony. As you may have guessed, this is not a real person, but a dreamy idealized vision of me which is much more fun to be inspired by.

What is that shimmery, magical version of yourself that you carry around in your head? Does she look like what you see in the mirror? Or does she dance around, just out of reach, until you give up and go for something more 'normal'.

I know for each of us there is our muse – that lady who lives her most elevated life and who we look to for inspiration.

I am blissfully happy with my quiet little life in New Zealand, almost as far away from Paris as you could hope to get, but that doesn't mean I can't be inspired by my chic French muse.

Listen to your muse

My muse inspires me to wear some classically French styles, yes, but also to do my own chic thing in my own way. I take her literally sometimes, and just the essence of her at others.

When I let her in, she switches on Carla Bruni music to play softly in the background. She makes me an omelette and salad for lunch. And she pours me a flute of sparkling mineral water when we sit down to relax before dinner.

She helps me be more playful with my clothing choices, and utterly feminine. She gives me gentle nudges when she can see that I am not honouring myself properly and encourages me to nestle in for a good night's sleep and forgo the sugar which doesn't support me.

She reminds me to paint my nails in a pretty shade each week. Clear red, summery coral or deep plum. She loves timeless colours and would faint in horror if I chose green, blue, or yellow. But that's her; what can I say. She's a classics girl.

She loves blue jeans, pearl stud earrings, a crisp white shirt, and a brightly coloured pair of ballet flats. She favours sheer pretty makeup and likes to move her body in a gentle and pleasurable way.

All of this to say, she is me. She is the me who knows what I am drawn to. She likes to see what is new for the season and choose from that if it takes her fancy, rather than be sold to.

And your muse is there too. Maybe she is French, and maybe she's not. She might be solidly you, or she might borrow from another culture, time in history, or lifestyle.

It is fun to identify your muse (or muses) and take inspiration from them as well as physical cues. Perhaps your muse is actually rather glam and goes to soirees in 1920s New York *a la* The Great Gatsby. You might have no need for ornate party frocks, but who says you can't wear a pair of chandelier earrings with jeans and a tee-shirt? Who says you can't cut your hair into the perfect flapper bob?

And aside from those things, it is fun to carry your muse around as a mindset, bringing her along to infuse levity into your day. I walk differently, converse with relaxed ease and have a tiny contented smile because I feel so good when she is with me.

I know you feel all these things too when you have your muse in mind.

Nostalgia as style inspiration

When you think about it, you may find, as I did, that the style you dream of has been with you for a long time. My Paris girl has been beguiling me since I was a teenager, and I still feel drawn to her with the same flutter now as I did then.

Look back at your past inspiration and enjoy the nostalgia of it. What lit you up as a little girl? What elements from then could you incorporate into your grown-up style now?

I find it comforting to bring in small parts of my younger years to the present day. It reminds me of the girl I was and encourages me to be forever young. To be playful and enjoy my life. It helps alleviate the seriousness of being an adult.

An example for me is that I adored pink, pretty, scented items. So, I enjoy wearing perfume, body mists, and fragranced lotions every day. When I buy something, I will see what the most feminine option is. My husband and I bought iPads at the same time last year to go on an overseas trip and I chose a gold tablet, with a flamingo pink cover. It looks so pretty, and I love that it is different to my husband's dark silver iPad with a dark charcoal cover.

Blend your loves

My favourite chic tip is to mix what you love together to create your own style, as well as inspire your direction in the future. Paris girl + feminine + bombshell = me. Others may love the classic Parisian style too, but tend more towards the rock chick, or bohemian perhaps.

When we give ourselves permission to love what we love, our own personal style blossoms beautifully. We don't need to worry if something is out of style or that we might feel silly articulating just *why* we love it. If we love it, that's enough.

And that's why it is so useful to consider Brian's zero-based thinking, because it weeds out choices that may have been made in a sensible and practical moment (how dull), or items that were given to us and aren't quite our style. We don't necessarily have to get rid of those 'offending' items, but it might help us choose differently in the future or look at ways to style something to be more to our muse's ideal taste.

Give yourself the gift of loving what you love and choosing what lights you up.

Your Chic Closet tips:

Consider whether the contents of your closet reveal the real you. Go and have a look right now and **see if you feel happy** with everything hanging in there.

Make some notes on **who your muse could be**. Is there a movie character you have always admired for their wardrobe? Write down all the details you remember and why you love them. When I brainstorm lists like this, surprising details pop out and I am inspired to start adding things into my wardrobe that completely lift everything else.

One example is that I love Coco Chanel's simple style, so I have collected inexpensive ropes of pearls, and layer them over a black top every so often. I always get compliments and I love the look.

Revisit **style genres that have intrigued you in the past** and note them down. Bring forward one or two details to the current day and enjoy playing around with them. Perhaps you adored glitter or blowing bubbles as a little girl. Can you start taking bubble baths? Buy a pretty phone cover? A writing pen with glitter floating around inside the barrel? Or what about a soft pink scarf for winter with fine fold threads woven through?

These gifts to your inner child will make her very happy indeed.

Chapter 2.
Fall in love with your current wardrobe

I am ashamed to admit this, but I probably take my wardrobe for granted a lot of the time. It is sometimes a seasonal thing where I forget that the weather is changing, and sometimes it is simply because I realize I haven't given my wardrobe any attention lately.

I might not have looked around to see what is out there nor been shopping for many months; or if I have bought new things, they were not intentional. Gaps can appear which prevent me from creating new outfits and I end up wearing the same few items over and over.

When this happens, I have my favourite ways to get excited about my wardrobe again. To kindle the style fire, I find it helpful to:

Borrow other people's enthusiasm

Nothing gets me more inspired about being fashionable and stylish than following fashion bloggers on Instagram or reading street style blogs. I think it is so cool that I can see what a well-dressed lady is wearing this very day in Paris or Milan. I love Instagram for this, by following accounts which appeal, and which inspire me to be more creative with my wardrobe. I sometimes look up hashtags too, such as #parisstreetstyle, #milanfashion or #ralphlaurenwomen for example. Whatever comes to mind I will have a look for and save my favourites. I come across new people to follow this way too.

Another excellent resource is Pinterest, and I enjoy pinning images I like onto my 'My Wardrobe' board. It is fun to look through it once I've gathered a few, because I can then see my favoured 'Fiona-style' emerging.

Re-organize everything

Without thinking about it too much (otherwise I will talk myself out of it and say it's too big of a job), I take everything out of my drawers and put them onto the bed. Then, sort and put back, seeing what I have as I go. Maybe I'll declutter a few pieces but it's more about reacquainting myself with what I have.

It is a nice surprise when you are excited to see items you've forgotten about (such as from the off-season that you are just coming into) and it's like they are brand new again. That's the best feeling, and means you have chosen well.

And it's the same with my hanging items, I take them all out of my closet and lay them on the bed and start with an empty rail. I put hangers back one by one, with my current favourites at the front. Anything I'm so-so about stays on the bed, and I either put it away if it's for the season we are not in, or if it is suitable for the current season, find out why don't I like it. I ask myself, 'Why do I avoid wearing this?'

There is a sense of relief I find, when I 'allow' myself to put an item into the donation box, when that garment was just hanging there, not bringing any joy into my life. I would rather someone else gets use from it, because I certainly am not.

Spend time in your closet

When I spend time in my closet organizing, mending, decluttering, playing around with new outfit combos, rearranging by colour, doing the seasonal switchover and all those kinds of things, I fall in love with my clothes again and feel satisfied with my choices. And, of course, if there are any gaps, I can easily identify them and shop with a purpose.

It's when I treat my closet as a dash-in-dash-out kind of situation that I feel dissatisfied and like I have nothing to wear. I don't take the time to get to know what I have and it's as if my clothes know that.

They feel unloved! I find this with so many areas in my life: the more love I give to that category, the more love I receive back.

Count your blessings

Start thinking of all the reasons why you are lucky to have your current wardrobe. Run a gratitude list in your mind going through the ways in which you are blessed in the clothing department. When I do this, it makes me feel better about everything and I can take inspired actions from there. At the very least, I feel happy and positive about the future.

I think to myself: *I am surrounded by my favourite colours. I love that my clothing is clean and comfortable. I have happy memories from these clothes. I have plenty of choice on any one day. I love to project my idealized 'French Chic' girl with these clothes. I have had the ability to buy them all. I am abundant in lovely clothing. I can wear anything I want from this selection. People in other countries would only wish to have all these clothes. I can dress up or dress down, formal, or casual. I have the freedom to dress how I please. I can have fun and play a part if I like, projecting power-lady; sexy chic; or cool and elegant. How lucky am I?*

Really, how could anyone feel uninspired after a gentle pep-talk like this?

Watch 'old favourite' fashion movies and programs

On a rainy and cozy day at home, I find it so soothing to watch a movie which reignites the love of style within me. *The Devil Wears Prada* is one such movie. It all starts with the opening credits, where beautiful New York women get ready for their day. Their underwear matches, they artfully apply makeup to their faces, choose pretty earrings, and slip into their high heels. (You can view this fab opening piece on YouTube by searching for 'opening montage the devil wears prada'.)

Watching this three-minute section motivates me to be my best, non-lazy self who makes an effort when she gets ready in the morning.

Plus, *The Devil Wears Prada* is humorous, which is just an added bonus. Laughing is so good for you and very much under-rated by some, I think. And near the end of the movie when they are in Paris? Swoon. It is such a beautiful and glamorous part of the movie and will make you want to do more with your wardrobe!

And a few more of my favourites?

Desperate Housewives. I like to re-watch episodes every now and then to be inspired by their homes (especially Bree and her Martha Stewart-ness), their slenderness and the way they dress. I would love to wear a pencil skirt and silk blouse like Bree does, but the reality is that I probably dress more casually like Susan, or maybe a mix of the two. And again, it is a really funny program.

Sex and the City. Both the series and the movies are wonderful. The girls have fun with fashion and inspire me to try different things in the way I dress. Plus, their apartments and closets are great to see, and being set in New York City is a definite bonus.

This is War. I love this movie because of Reece Witherspoon's personal style in it. The outfits are great – very wearable – and good to take inspiration from. I love her casual look of skinny jeans, high heels, and a cute top. Your man won't mind watching this one with you either, because it's quite an action/boy/comedy movie.

Wardrobe malaise can set in at any time, and often will sneak up on you. Maybe it's the middle of the season and you are sick of your clothes. It's easy to be excited about the changing season and the promise of different outfits, but once you're a few months in, everything seems a bit samey.

Or you've just been ignoring your personal style for a while. Whatever the reason, I wish you all the best as you rekindle your passion with these tips!

Your Chic Closet tip:

Choose an angle that most excites your emotions, and **do something towards it, even if tiny, right now**. Anything I've ever done on the spur of the moment, whether it's reorganizing my hanging items by colour or in complete outfits, or deciding to recreate a look from Pinterest, I've been thrilled with the results. Strike while the iron is hot, chic friend; it's a popular saying for good reason.

Chapter 3.
Develop your style with a personal brand

You might think that because you aren't in business you don't have a personal brand, but you do; we all do, whether it is intentional or not.

Designing your own personal style is simply you offering a consistent and understandable message to others. The colours and styles you wear, and how you present yourself to the world all gather together to create *marque toi* (or 'Brand YOU').

People will get what you're about when you are consistent in all areas of your life. In addition, *you* will trust yourself, because you will feel less of a fraud than if you were one way in public and another way in private. An extreme case could be someone who is impeccably turned out when you see them, yet at home dresses in stained yoga pants with hair like a bird's nest.

It's enlightening to consider what your 'brand' might look like, and this inspires easy ways in which to add more of what you love into your closet. In this chapter you will find twelve of my favourite ways to effortlessly add to your *marque toi*, and give yourself and those in your life the sense of safety and constancy that this cohesiveness provides.

The best thing though, is that all of these points are just plain fun to do as well. I always find that life is elevated when I'm a little bit playful and not too serious. That's when my best ideas come out, such as tying a scarf to my bag handle (when I've not touched my scarves for months), or wearing two items together that I don't normally pair.

There really is so much that we can do by combining our current wardrobe with a newly inspired state of mind. I hope you enjoy going through these questions and noting down ideas as they bubble up.

Find a fresh journal, or open a new page on your computer or phone and start writing down what you love by pondering the questions below. If you keep everything in one place, you will look back on your pages of answers with such fondness, and new angles will be sparked whenever you read or add to these notes.

Let's get started!

1. What are your absolute favourite colours to surround yourself with, both in clothing and at home? Don't just write down blue, write down all the nuances of blue that you love: duck egg, periwinkle, deep sea blue, the colour of the sky at dusk... I am energized by choosing evocative names of the shades I adore, such as vanilla, blush pink and pale buttercream yellow. Keep this list to inspire future purchases and colour combination ideas.

2. How can you imagine your closet feeling? Then, how would you change your closet to reflect this feeling? Is there something easy you can do straight away? For me, I wanted a feminine, elegant and beautifully simple place to dress. An easy step I took was to straighten things up, and arrange clothes in a different way than they had been (by colour, or tops then bottoms, or by seasons etc).

3. If you could start your wardrobe from scratch, what kind of image would you love to project? I'd go for a chic, classic, slightly sexy wardrobe. Think fitted jeans, high pumps and a Chanel jacket or nipped-waist blazer. This brings to mind an Emmanuelle Alt style. Why not start to incorporate elements of *your* dream style into your life using items you already own? Doing this means you will (literally) be stepping into the new you, the one who is aligned with your

desired personal style. With my imagined outfit above, I already owned all those pieces, but I very rarely wore them all together. Of course I do now, once I put the puzzle pieces together!

4. Start a Pinterest file of idealized, maybe slightly over-the-top looks that you love, so you can be inspired when creating your look. Once you have a few saved you may notice a theme emerging. Ask yourself what it is about each outfit that appeals. You will then have a topline guide for your own evolving style.

5. What inspires you? For me, even though I love the countryside to live in, I feel most inspired by big cities such as New York and Paris; apartment living with elevators; sipping a cocktail in fancy hotel lobby bars; and department stores. I love to imagine I am that city girl and dress accordingly.

6. Make a list of your favourite brands and tease out what you love about them. Are there elements in your lists that you could use to dress yourself? Brands that appeal to me are Starbucks, Estee Lauder/Aerin Lauder, *Victoria* magazine, Ralph Lauren, and Martha Stewart. I love their elegance, femininity, originality, sense of history, living life creatively and making everything around them beautiful, even the utilitarian things. From these examples I get

a feeling for the kinds of clothes I want to wear (feminine and elegant, even with my casual style) and how I go about that (I love the 'make do and mend' philosophy, so I regularly repair items, or even upcycle by patching denim etc).

7. Get yourself out of your everyday surroundings to brainstorm ideas for your ideal personal style. Add 30-60 minutes to an errand trip so you can journal inspiration at a nice café (even though you could do it at home with a coffee for free) or go to the beach, mountains or a public park. People-watch, daydream, and let ideas flow.

8. Deep down, what have you always imagined yourself wearing and thought it would be just a fantasy? Dare to dream big! I have always loved the Chanel suit. A few years ago, I bought a cream-coloured Chanel-inspired tweed jacket from Zara, and feel great wearing it with jeans, or a simple pair of black pants. And before that even, I bought a large piece of black-and-white houndstooth fabric in nubby silk, and would love to have it made into a knee-length skirt and jacket. Ideally by me, but more likely by a tailor. The Chanel suit might not be in my budget, but there are other ways to get the look. What looks do you love that you could get in different ways?

9. Have a one-week personal focus where you choose an aspect of your look to give your energy

and attention to. Perhaps you might choose to wear a bit more makeup than you usually do, and enjoy applying it each morning. You might not want to commit to doing this forever more, but having a focus on one aspect of your personal style for just a week is a fun way to explore things. Other ideas could be wearing more colour in your clothing, accessorizing each day, doing your hair in a different style, or polishing your nails and keeping them maintained for the week. Some of these 'chic habits' you might carry on with, and some you might be happy to try once then leave behind.

10. When building your personal style, dress for *you*. Yes, I certainly take note of when I am complimented on an outfit or a colour I am wearing, and when my husband says he loves my smoky-eye makeup, but I also do all of these things for me. I enjoy expressing my desired self by choosing my look each day. Go with what you love and you really can't go wrong, it's as simple as that.

11. List 10-20 words that reflect how you want to show up and what it is you want your look to 'feel' like. Put each word into Pinterest one at a time. From the images that come up, pin five for each word and save to a board called something like My Style Essence, My Personal Style, Style Essence Words or similar – something that feels

good to you. Then, only pin images which give you that YES! feeling straight away, and, here's the secret trick: do it quickly and without thinking about it too much. Pin, pin, pin, pin, pin and onto the next word. When you go back to that board afterwards, it should give you a spine-tinglingly good visual representation of your personal style to inspire new ideas to try.

12. What signature touch could you add to your look? Think of Coco Chanel with the camellia flower she used symbolically, and as a buttonhole decoration on her jackets and dresses. She also had the lion symbol (since she was born under the astrological sign of Leo) which she used in different areas of her life. In addition, Coco had a strong colour palette of black and white that she often used (and it's the two shades used in her makeup packaging now). What could your signature touches be?

Let this exploration of your personal brand be *fun*. Think about what uplifts you and makes you happy. Think about what you want the essence of your personal style to feel like, then create it day-by-day to show the world who you are.

Your Chic Closet Tips:

Know that **you don't have to create your personal style all in one hit**, but it's a good thing to keep in mind so you can polish it over time. Ask yourself of a decision, 'Does this fit in with my ideal view of myself?' or, 'Am I aligned with my personal brand right now?'

Your personal style will always be evolving (as will you). Where you start out is not where you will finish, so don't be afraid to make it feel right for you *in this moment*. Put your ideas into action and refine your look over time. You will become more 'you' by doing this, and you will also enjoy playing around with your look for the rest of your life. Imagine still being excited by your style as an 85-year old! Wouldn't that be wonderful?

Chapter 4.
Cultivating the 'expensive' look

I love thinking about the concept of dressing yourself in a way that conveys wealth and class in an old-fashioned sense. Of course, money is no guarantee to looking good. As we all know, extremely rich people can still look cheap. There are plenty of walking testimonies, celebrity or otherwise, that show you can look tacky even having spent plenty.

And there are those without much money but with an innate sense of their own style who can look fabulously upmarket whatever they wear. Those are the ones I want to emulate. So what are those elusive elements that makes someone look quietly expensive?

Firstly, colour plays a big part. To me, **expensive colours are neutrals**, worn together. Think of a whole outfit in tones of caramel and cream. Black with off-white, or black and caramel are very stylish too. In general: black, navy, winter white, beige or caramel, and red.

I would also add soft, muted tones of blush pink, sea-foam green, Tiffany blue and other such shades depending on what suits your colouring. Neon brights don't feel luxurious or wealthy to me, especially when paired with black. I remember hearing once that putting black with a bright colour makes both look cheap.

But colour is a deeply personal thing, and it also depends on your skin tone what flatters you best. Darker skin can look chic and sophisticated in bright colours, whereas they overpower me, so consider your colouring when you are choosing the shades in your 'wealthy woman' palette.

Fabric-wise, I always think **woven cloth, or structured knits look more expensive**. Going the other way are floppy t-shirt knits and floaty garments. Again, this is my personal taste in clothing coming through, but I always feel more pulled together in a tailored blazer or semi-fitted dress with simple lines. And what I have noticed in my observations of those who dress 'rich', there are more woven fabrics than knits in general.

Wearing classic styles whispers money to me. Luckily I love the classics and never feel more at home than in a well-cut pair of jeans and a white shirt (in my imagination this is 'the Hamptons look'), or in tailored black pants and a tuxedo front shirt, with high heels if dressing up. Without fail I always feel affluent in my classic clothing.

Shoe-wise, I love the classics too – the black leather ballet flat, and white or navy canvas low-top sneakers. A perfectly pointed stiletto heel never goes out of fashion. I always think chunky heels make a leg look chunky, even on skinny starlets. Wedges, ditto, but there are some cute wedges out there that are finer, not so extreme, that look pretty and well-bred, and are very useful in summer.

Consider where you are going to. When I visit a dear friend in an old money part of town, I love dressing up in my most classic outfits, clothing I imagine I might wear if I lived there.

There is nothing I enjoy more (after dressing up) than taking a stroll around the shops, maybe trying on some clothing or just having a look through the stores in fancy areas. I notice the outfits and details that others are wearing. There is a different vibe in wealthy areas. I like to absorb it and take it home with me. Funnily enough I am more interested in how older ladies dress in these areas; I find their style fascinating.

Wearing big sunglasses imparts an air of mystery and glamour. I like to keep my favourite pairs polished, and wear them every day. Plus, they protect your eyes from the sun, which is important for both the eyes themselves, and preventing wrinkles. I adore aviators too; they look very luxe and jet-set to me.

You don't need an expensive bag, so don't worry if a designer bag is out of your budget, but **make sure your bag is tidy and clean**, and still has its shape. Purchasing a classic style and looking after it will go a long way towards contributing to your expensive look.

I have my eye on a Louis Vuitton shoulder bag for my upcoming 50th birthday and, while my head has been turned by a quirky statement piece, I will more likely go for a classic style which I will be able to wear for decades to come, and is also less expensive than the trendier styles.

Attending to **grooming is *très* important** and vital to looking chic. I always love to be well-groomed even when at home by myself, and especially when I go out. I have been perfecting my grooming regime over time, and by making myself do it even when I couldn't be bothered it has now become a habit, much like brushing my teeth, so I do it automatically.

I exfoliate and shave my legs in the shower every two days and wash my hair every second day on the alternate days, so I don't spend too long in the shower. I apply body lotion every single morning to every part of my body that I can reach. I love wearing fragranced body lotions; even if they don't match my perfume, as long as they are from the same 'scent family', they layer together with my other body products to create a lasting fragrance.

I always wear perfume, even on a home day. I wear it for me, so I am never without it. I enjoy having a variety to choose from. I still love my Chanel No. 5, and more recently Chanel Coco Noir (which is softer than you would think), however I have a wardrobe of inexpensive fragrances for everyday wear.

Polished nails suggest you have plenty of time to lounge around being tended to, but they also show that you take care of yourself. I always do my toes in the summer (I mostly give them a break in winter), and I do my own fingernails every week.

My preferred look is to keep them short (level with the end of my finger), in a bright crème colour, such as classic red, tangerine or plum. I also have pale pink and sheer beige, but enjoy having a coloured nail mostly (however, I suspect the old money crowd prefers nude pink, like the English royal ladies do).

Having short, painted nails is both a modern look, plus it is practical. With short nails, I can go most of the week without having to touch up any chips.

For makeup, the wealthy look is ***le no makeup look***. A polished, natural glow, and a little bronzer. Being so fair, I always look for a bronzer which has a yellow tint versus orange. Or else I go the peaches and cream route with a tiny amount of foundation, a dusting of translucent powder, pinky blush and glossy lips. Groomed brows, eyeliner and mascara completes my look. When I want more drama, I amp up the eye makeup.

Lastly is jewellery. Sure, being draped in diamonds might seem like 'the rich look', but I actually think having **a few special pieces gives off an aura of wealth**. You will notice that old money ladies will often wear understated jewellery such as a slim gold wedding band and simple stud earrings.

My nana gave me a pair of cultured pearl stud earrings for my fourteenth birthday and I have worn them regularly for the past thirty-five years! They have transcended all fashion trends for me and make me feel fresh and elegant. And they weren't expensive either as my nana wasn't a rich lady, but she always favoured quality.

Keeping real jewellery clean ensures that it sparkles and gives off a wealthy look too. If you don't have jewellery cleaning solution, dishwashing liquid, hot water and a clean toothbrush will make anything look beautiful. Use on gold and all precious stones except for emeralds.

I squirt a tiny amount of dishwash onto the toothbrush, clean my ring or necklace carefully (including the chain), then rinse in warm water and dry. You will be amazed how good your pieces look when you do this. Never clean pearls this way though. They just need a polish with a soft cloth and plenty of wear, as the oils in your skin keep them shiny.

Actually, '**clean**' is probably is one of the most underrated tips in looking expensive. Think pristine clothing – in good repair with no stains, holes, or missing buttons; just-washed bouncy hair; sparkling jewellery; polished, well-cared-for shoes; and a handbag that is in good condition, with no tatty or broken bits. Yes, some maintenance costs, but you can do a lot for free and make low-cost items look more expensive than they really are. I love that! More dash than cash!

Your Chic Closet Tips:

How seriously you take this chapter is up to you. You might not aspire to look 'rich', but it's intriguing to ponder the aesthetics of a wealthy look. I combine 'rich lady' style principles together with what I am drawn to, to make 'my' look.

And so it is with you, combining your favourite influences together to create your own inimitable style. If dressing to look wealthy appeals to you, why not **combine some of the tips in this chapter with your own preferred personal style**. Be boho and fastidiously well turned out. Millennial chic with classic tailoring. Have fun mixing and matching!

Chapter 5.
Inject excitement with a capsule du mois

There is plenty of talk around of capsule collections, with closet look books and also limiting your wardrobes to a certain number. Jennifer L. Scott of *Madame Chic* fame has her 10-item wardrobe (plus extras) which she assembles each season. Courtney Carver has *Project 333* where she recommends choosing 33 items (including accessories and outerwear) to wear for three months.

My good friend and author Kristi Belle, is very good at curating a tiny closet, but for me, I'd be too scared to get rid of everything like she does. She really is fearless!

Just the other day I was feeling like my day-to-day wardrobe needed a little oomph. In the old days I would have gone out and bought something new.

This was when I spent a lot, always seemed to be paying off my credit card, and decluttered regularly because my closet was 'inexplicably' stuffed full to the brim.

Instead, I did something I have found works well, and that is to inject excitement into my current closet by pulling together collections as and when I feel called to. On impulse, I decided to choose my favourite twenty-one pieces that would make an attractive, comfortable, appropriate and stylish capsule to wear right now.

I chose the number 21 for a couple of reasons. It is the in-between of the above ladies' recommended numbers and I thought it was a good easy way not to have extras or include accessories, and it also happens to be the day of the month I was born, so I have a natural affinity with this number. My lucky 21.

I purposely kept the thought process simple, and chose as quickly as possible. It always works well for me to do something fast. I like to see just how fast I can get things done, otherwise I tend to dawdle, fall into perfectionism and eventually lose interest because I'm not getting anything achieved.

Within five minutes I had chosen my favoured capsule *du mois* ('of the month' – I wanted to put capsule *du jour* because it sounds fun, but 'of the day' is not a very long time to wear everything in my capsule).

I started with the pieces I had been wearing on non-stop rotation (literally a handful of items) and added in others that I knew fit me well, I enjoyed wearing, and were appropriate for the current season and how I spend my days.

Hang *everything*

The detail that really makes this the most appealing way to increase your wardrobe's allure, is to clear a space on your hanging rail. I do this by pushing out-of-season items further along the bar, or hang them somewhere else. I then have a nice open space in which to hang my selection, and I hang everything I've chosen. Even tee-shirts and knit items.

This one little detail makes all the difference to the enjoyment of my capsule. It's like my own *petite* boutique where everything is hanging together, showing me what goes with what, and displaying the colour palette I have chosen. If I don't wear items very often or won't be wearing them until the next season, I'll fold them away in a drawer or on a shelf. But since my 21-piece collection is going to be worn frequently, there won't be time for knit items to develop shoulder-marks from hangers.

Think about a clothing store – most of the time everything is hanging up, even quite delicate items, or pieces that you might think would be better stored folded. And that's so that customers can visualize items together, pick the hanger up and hold the clothing item against themselves, and see how all the colours harmonize together.

I started hanging all my current season clothes

many years ago, and I've never stopped, because it makes a huge difference to how easy it is to get dressed in the morning, and I don't forget about anything I own.

Things that I still keep in drawers are gym clothes, underwear, loungewear, and socks etc. But with my dressier knit tops or brand-new tee-shirts that are for everyday wear, they will be hung with my jeans, pants and dresses.

Not just seasonal

Creating a mini-capsule collection is also a great idea if you are wanting to lose some weight. I know the stress that comes when you feel like *everything* is too tight on you, and that stress has you eating to soothe yourself which you know is not going to help the issue, but you just can't stop!

What has been helpful to me is to go through my closet and find everything that will fit my current size (even if it's slightly 'too good' for everyday wear; maybe not a ball gown, but, say, a dressy top or pair of trousers).

Hang all of those items together front-and-centre in your closet and enjoy wearing them. I found that it was such a relief to have items which fit comfortably and, with my dressier clothes included (because I didn't have much that fit me well at that time), my options were extended. I also felt good because I was wearing my 'best' clothes as well.

Why not wear your silky blouse with a pussy-cat

bow to the supermarket with jeans and ballet flats? You may feel a little conspicuous at the time, but when someone says how nice you look, you realize it's not a bad thing to be slightly over-dressed. And for me I only felt over-dressed because I wore such casual clothes most of the time. Maybe I needed the push to dress better?

(I expand on this concept in an upcoming chapter: Chapter 11. 'Inspiring yourself to slim with your wardrobe'.)

The past few weeks I have worn a blazer more often, and even though my outfit underneath is not that different to what I would normally wear, I have had multiple comments along the lines of, 'Why so dressed up?' and 'You look nice. What's the occasion?' It was only the addition of a blazer – so easy to do! Plus, just what am I saving my better clothes for? A rainy day? My old age? This really confirmed to me that I would do well to enjoy my clothes regularly – *all* of them. And the blazer was in my consciousness because I had put it in my current collection, to round out the look of my choices.

When you design a capsule collection, the real fun is when you come to get dressed the next morning. It felt like I was browsing in *Boutique Fifi*, and I can tell you, it is a very stylish place to shop. Plus, I haven't spent any money either.

Creating a capsule from your existing wardrobe has a magic all of its own, that's for sure.

Your Chic Closet tips:

Work out a number and method of creating a capsule collection that works well for you. It all depends on how often you do your laundry, whether you feel more comfortable with fewer or more items to choose from, and what you have in your wardrobe to start with.

Then, go straight to your closet and start gathering items for your collection. Go quickly, be decisive and **stop when you get to your chosen number**. Take a look back over your choices and see what you think. Is it sufficiently exciting for you?

If you go over or under slightly it doesn't matter. It's only an arbitrary number after all, but the times I've done this, it has been fascinating that as I get to the end of my clothes to choose from, the number adds up perfectly. As in, I don't get half-way through my clothes and find I've gotten up to 21. And I also found that I had a good mix of dresses, pants, tops and jackets.

Your inner stylist knows what she is doing, so call on her services. She will be thrilled to hear from you.

Chapter 6.
Claiming 'sexiness' as a state of mind

One of my favourite questions to ask myself when I am journaling inspiration is, 'What excites me right now?' or, 'What would make me happy?' Also, 'What would I love to do if I wasn't thinking of anyone else's opinion?' I mix everything in my life together – both writing and home related things, and I also like to do this with my wardrobe and the way in which I dress.

In a recent happy-list I mentioned travelling to Paris, and also of having a sexier vibe to my personal style. Now, I don't think I will be flying to Paris in the next little while, but I am deciding to claim sexy as a state of mind. It's an underlying sexiness though. I don't desire to dress tarty or wear super-short skirts or flaunt massive cleavage (but if you love this, then please go for it!), but to choose sexiness as more of an internal chic radar.

Having an inner sexiness kills off frump and helps me when I am making decisions – anything from clothes shopping to how we decorate our home. When I bought high heels recently, they had to be sexy. You see, I hadn't bought nice going-out shoes for a long time, and even those were a bit frumpy. My husband Paul said to me, 'You've got to go and buy some nice shoes!' But I'd think, 'Well we hardly go out anywhere, I'm being thrifty wearing what I've got'. But no more, that was the old me. The new me chooses to have a sexy state of mind. Even *one* pair of glamorous shoes can make a difference.

(Please note when I am talking of buying glamorous and sexy high heels, I am *not* talking about expensive towering shoes that are a danger to walk in. The heels I chose were the right height for me, and within my budget!)

I remember a conversation between two customers that I had the good fortune to be near, when I was working in our shoe store before we sold it. The situation was this. A kindly local mum brought in a French woman whose daughter was just starting at the same school as her child, as they had only moved to New Zealand three weeks previous.

While the daughter was trying on school shoes, the two women were looking at ladies' shoes and pointing out the styles they liked. 'Oh, I don't wear heels anymore, I live in flats', said the Kiwi mum, who was very practically dressed. 'Why is that, why do you not wear heels?' asked the French woman, in her musical accent. 'If you buy good quality, they will be comfortable, no?'

Of course, the French woman with her charming accent said the word 'quality' with the emphasis on the last syllable to make it sound quite lilting. I could have listened to her all day.

Now please don't think I am judging the lady from New Zealand, as she was dressed just as many other women around here do, very normal. But I took notice of what the French mother was wearing. She had on slim-cut jeans tucked into brown leather boots that had a slight heel (I would guess between 2-3 inches at most, maybe lower), but still appropriate for a casual weekend look, a pretty top and hair cut in that uniquely French tousled way. She wasn't wearing tons of makeup, jewellery or bling, but she looked fresh, pretty and appropriate.

I was so tickled by this chic sighting. The French woman was genuinely perplexed as to why the other mother had stopped wearing heels. It was almost as if the Kiwi lady had told her she'd given up on life! And both these ladies looked to be only in their thirties, I would say.

I still do wear a lot of flat shoes and very low heels (that are virtually flats), but I also remember this French woman's advice when I am looking at shoes. Thanks to her I have some higher but still wearable sandals and alternate these with my ballet flats in the summer. I have a pair of cork wedges which are very wearable for an everyday summer sandal too.

And I have a few pairs of winter ankle boots with

slightly higher heels than I might have chosen. It seems that with boots your feet are completely 'wrapped' and therefore you can feel quite stable in heels. I also love the man-tailoring look of a lace-up brogue with a heel. So chic.

I hope you can see in this chapter that you don't need to have an all or nothing mindset. You don't need to be either sexy *or* frumpy, wear skyscraper heels *or* complete flats. By adopting an inner sexiness and going for comfortable lower heels, you can feel elegant and stylish within your happy constraints. There is no need for discomfort, either physically or in how you present yourself.

And many thanks to my French 'sister' for her wise and stylish advice!

Your Chic Closet Tips:

Could you use this French lady's advice as well? **Do you have a pair of heels that make you feel good** (low or otherwise)? Of course there might be medical issues that bar you from anything but flats, but for me, it was just never-thinking-about-it combined with a dash of laziness.

There is something fun about not being entirely practical, don't you think?

And please do join me in claiming **sexiness as an inner state of being**. It's a game changer.

Chapter 7.
Creating your own fashion uniform

Have you noticed that the top fashion designers and editors wear their own uniform of sorts?

No matter what is happening on the runway, Michael Kors is there in his black top and aviators. In the documentary *The September Issue*, I couldn't help but notice Anna Wintour dressed in the same silhouette each day – fitted bodice dress with a little gathered skirt, tiny fine-knit cardigan, and chunky beads.

Giorgio Armani is famous for wearing a black or navy t-shirt and black trousers. French Vogue editor Emmanuelle Alt wears her uniform all the time – skinny leg cropped trousers with a trim-cut blazer and heels. And I mostly see Ralph Lauren in jeans and a white or denim shirt with Western boots, or if he really wants to dress it up, he puts on a tuxedo jacket.

Perhaps their version of a fashion uniform might be a colour. The late Sonia Rykiel was known for her combination of flaming red hair, smoky eye makeup and perpetual look of black, black and more black.

If you care to google-image just about anyone high up in the fashion world, you'll notice a lot of their photos look very similar. Of course there will be those who wear something cutting edge and different every day, but I believe they are the exception rather than the rule.

They are obviously onto something, and they're doing it without telling us!

What they're telling us is to look to the trends each season, but what they're doing is wearing simple and classic shapes that suit their body and are comfortable to wear, and make them feel like themselves.

Rather than look to the models and fashion pages for inspiration, I actually prefer to take note of what the tastemakers are wearing. This observation makes me feel better about choosing to have a small wardrobe of simple classics, and looking to refine it even more over time.

I love this fabulous quote from Giorgio Armani:

"At every age, what makes you have a great sense of style is the ability to listen to your own instincts and to choose what makes you feel comfortable and confident. Being elegant is not a matter of age but of attitude."

I think as we get older, we are more drawn to the idea of a uniform: our best 'go-to' outfits. It is something that naturally evolves over time, because we have worked out what looks best on our body. In addition, as we age we may no longer care so much about what others think of us. We dress to please ourselves and wear the items that make us most happy.

Many of us want a simpler life too, and having a go-to outfit or style makes it much easier to get dressed in the morning. Barack Obama wore only two colours of suits in the White House and counted it as the secret to his high productivity. He told Vanity Fair: "You'll see I wear only grey or blue suits. I'm trying to pare down decisions. I don't want to make decisions about what I'm eating or wearing. Because I have too many other decisions to make."

The great thing about curating your own fashion uniform is that you can make life easier, but still have fun too. I have the clothing items and shapes that suit me and my lifestyle, and I also add in colour and texture with my footwear, handbag and accessories such as scarves and jewellery.

Seasonal uniforms

Your uniform may change seasonally as well. I love skinny jeans and a crisply pressed shirt in the spring or autumn, and skinny jeans with a fine-knit jumper in the winter. When it's just too warm for jeans in the summer, I switch to dresses, which suit my body type more than skirts.

When I was working out what I best like to wear each season, I wrote down my options, because it seemed like I always forgot from one year to the next and would be stuck with a changing season and no clue what to wear!

When I came up with these principles for myself, gosh, it made life so much easier. (They weren't so prescriptive that I felt trapped in one style, rather, they were guidelines that I knew worked for me.)

Before I came to these conclusions, it was almost painful to change seasons. I would cling on to the outfits I had been wearing, but become too hot (or cold) once the weather started changing. That's when I saw that I needed to come up with my seasonal uniforms, that I could easily change up with accessories.

Do your homework

It seems like an obscenely luxurious thing to do when others are simply getting through their day , but when you take the time to work out what looks and feels good on you, flatters your figure, suits your lifestyle and budget, and then fill in the gaps of what is missing, it makes your life so much calmer and more enjoyable.

You do the thinking a few times a year (to ensure you don't fall into a style rut, and to accommodate that your body might be changing over time too) and then you can forget about it.

In the end, I think it's a balance of feeling

comfortable in what you are wearing and knowing that it flatters your figure type and colouring, and not slipping into a boring, predictable way of dressing.

How I like to use fashion is to see what pops out at me each season, and infuse a freshness into my wardrobe this way. It might be a colour that I fall in love with, such as melon or Kelly green. Or I might decide to add a pair of boyfriend jeans to my staple diet of skinny jeans.

And of course, accessories are a simple and (sometimes) inexpensive way to zing up a go-to look. Oversized sunglasses for a sexy allure, a new brightly coloured matte lipstick instead of the usual nude gloss, or trying a voluminous fine-cotton scarf instead of the classic silk square.

It's all about the mix, and for me it's nice not to take fashion too seriously so that I can dress in a simple, classic and easy way most of the time, and step it up when I am in the mood to stand out more.

You get to decide how 'strict' your uniform is too, from variations of the same outfit every day, to knowing what silhouettes and colours you prefer and dressing from there. As detailed in Chapter 3. 'Develop your style with a personal brand', by choosing pieces which reflect your personality, you give a sense of cohesion to those around you, directly or indirectly. People feel that they know you.

And far from feeling constrained, it's incredible the sense of freedom you can feel when choosing to keep your personal style very simple and recognizable. For some, fashion is a constant exploration of new ideas, but for many of us, developing our own fashion uniform means we can enjoy getting dressed in the morning knowing we will look good.

Your Chic Closet Tips:

Consider if you already have a kind of uniform without realizing it (you probably do). If so, it will likely be silhouettes, colours and styles that flatter you the most. Pinpoint what these are, and build on your best looks when you are shopping for new clothes, or putting outfits together with your existing wardrobe.

Make it fun, rather than a limiting way of dressing. Branch out with new details when you want to, and also feel soothed that you have the comfort of your 'uniform'. It's the best of both worlds really!

Chapter 8.
Decluttering your closet with inspiration

In my experience, a major roadblock on the path to living your chicest life is being surrounded by too many possessions, and the wrong kind of possessions for you. Even for those of us who are constantly editing our surroundings by being intentional with the kind of home and personal style we want, well, there are still areas that we'd love to feel better.

The changing of the main seasons twice a year is a perfect time to dive into your wardrobe. In the Spring, I am excited about washing my merino woollens, sorting out what I want to keep for next year and making a pile to donate that I haven't worn much and always seem to find a reason not to. There are so many variables - the colour's not quite right, the shape isn't good for you or the feel of the fabric doesn't make your skin happy.

And sometimes, it's just that an item doesn't look as good as it used to. When something is a favourite it's hard to let go of, but then when you think about how often you've worn it (a lot), you can probably admit that you've had your money's worth. I came across a great quote on a blog (which is no longer there, sadly) which helps me release items from my closet:

*"Last season, I gave away my favourite navy and white blouse. It was worn out looking, and **I could no longer wear it with confidence as a best quality item in my wardrobe**."*

The last part of this quote which I have bolded, helps me immensely when I am dithering over decluttering something.

In my dream quest for a perfectly curated clothing collection, I enjoy editing out the not-quite-right pieces and this allows all my favourites and newer items to shine brightly, making me happy when I slide open the wardrobe door (or dresser drawer) in the morning. I do this year-round and keep a donation box in our guest bedroom which gathers up saleable items and is donated when full.

To inspire and keep me focused on my wardrobe journey, I have imagined a scenario to keep in mind what I want my wardrobe to have the essence of.

You are in the shining city of Paris. It's your first day there and you've emerged from your darling little hotel room, showered and fresh, with shiny clean blow-dried hair and light, glowing makeup. You are meeting a dear friend for lunch later on, but the morning is all yours.

Taking care to keep track of the streets and alleys as you look around the arrondissement you are in, you turn into a quaint cobbled side street and look in a boutique window. As you walk in your eyes are immediately assaulted with racks and racks of mismatched clothing in all different sizes and colours.

You have a hard time imagining that an outfit can be pulled from all these racks despite a plethora of clothing styles and many, many pieces to choose from. There are shoeboxes stacked up in uneven piles everywhere and other unrelated items for sale also.

Because the boutique is so packed with stock, it can't easily be cleaned and this lends to its overall sense of stagnation and mustiness. The music being played adds to your 'get me outta here' feeling - you literally have trouble breathing easily with all this happening around you.

You exit the boutique quickly and look at the next one you pass. Aaah, that looks more inviting.

A gleaming black and glass front door is flanked by potted standard buxus trees and it shuts behind you as you step across the polished white ash floor and onto a huge, Persian silk rug in shades of black, grey, taupe and cream. The rug is faded and almost threadbare but it looks amazing, and absolutely perfect in this setting.

'Bonjour Madame', the slender shop assistant calls out melodically from her counter.

Right in front of you is a large round oak table with an oversized vase of fragrant white and pale pink lilies in the centre, and glossy books, beautiful candles, artisanal soaps, and tubes of handcream arranged around it.

You notice the soft level of sultry jazz lounge music playing at a slow tempo which lulls you into a relaxing frame of mind.

As you look around you see there aren't a great deal of items for sale in this store, but everything in there you would happily have in your own wardrobe. It's like someone has curated the most perfect and deceptively simple capsule collection in expensive-looking muted tones and chic neutrals, and you are in love with it all.

I've often daydreamed about having a wardrobe that is like a *bijou* and chic Parisian boutique and why shouldn't it be a reality for me? Why do I need to hold onto everything I've ever owned? Pieces I'll never wear again and items in different sizes, just because I've spent money on them?

Do I want my closet to resemble that first store?

Isn't it better that all of those things go to someone

else who will enjoy wearing them if I'm never going to?

I now choose to keep things quite minimal as I can't stand digging through clothes I've grown tired of, never really liked, or pieces which don't fit me correctly anymore. When it comes to clothing, I am not sentimental.

I love to pare down to the most perfectly distilled (yet ever evolving) wardrobe which means I can think less about what to put on in the morning, because I've already put time and energy into planning it before then.

Keeping the vision of my perfect Parisian boutique is my main inspiration. I wonder what you can see in your boutique? Visualizing little scenarios is a soothing way to drift off to sleep at night, and stepping into your ideal boutique could be a fun one.

It might be up a tiny cobbled street in Paris, like mine, or you might imagine yourself stepping into a luxurious London department store. Or what about a co-op of one-of-a-kind hand-spun and knitted wool items? Or a 1950s vintage store? Your choices are endless. Find the boutique that is perfect for you, and come on inside.

Your Chic Closet Tips:

Start noticing what you consistently push aside in your closet. Why don't you wear these things? At the end of the season, if you haven't wanted to wear them yet again, why not consider donating (or selling)? Start with one or two items that you know you'll never want to wear again if you are nervous about making a mistake.

Or, a tip that I love, is to **take everything out of your wardrobe and *only* put back the absolute yesses**. See how enticing your selection looks and box up the rest. Put them somewhere else to 'mature' while you think about it. Then, in a month or so have a look. You might take out a few items, but you may also be pleasantly surprised that you are happy to release the rest to be worn and loved by someone else.

Chapter 9.
The spiritual aspect to looking after your clothes

Like anyone, I mostly take good care of my clothing, but there have also been times when I have been a bit lazy and not looked after things as well as I could.

At those times I'd just stuff clothes in my closet and only think to do laundry when my husband said he had no underwear left. Don't laugh, it has happened a few times recently because I've been so focused on my writing. And yes, I know, some of you might say, "Well he knows where the machine is", but I am at home full-time and he works five to six days a week, and they are long workdays too. So, I am in charge of laundry management currently, but sometimes I do let things slide!

What I have found, from getting and keeping my washing up-to-date, is that looking after my clothes and accessories has paid more dividends than I realized. Here is my process, detailing all the extra steps I do when I am taking care of my 'investments' (after all, I have spent hard-earned money on my clothes and want them to last as long as possible).

- Notice that I haven't washed clothes for a few days and there are quite a few items in the laundry hamper.

- Separate into light and dark washes, check for areas to spot clean, wash, and hang on the line when loads are finished.

- Iron shirts while damp from the washing machine and dry on hangers with the top button done up (it's so much easier than ironing a dry shirt and I don't have to muck around with the steam setting on my iron and putting water into it – yes, I am lazy).

- Tidy up my closet, and restore order by putting things where they should be.

- Fold and put away clothing when dry, check for any areas to mend.

- Lint-shave any items that are showing pilling.

- Snip off loose threads and annoying labels.

- Mend tiny holes if possible.

- Swap over warm- and cool-weather clothing twice a year.

- Check if clothing is still good and downgrading when appropriate. (From best/going out, to home wear, to the rag bag.) Donate anything that I don't want to wear or doesn't project the image I see for myself (I don't do this as often as I used to because I am much more selective when shopping now, but mistakes do happen, or perhaps I have been given something).

- Clean and/or polish shoes, check if they need resoling or any repairs.

- Tidy up the shoe wardrobe – take all shoes out, dust off shelves, and replace shoes neatly with current season footwear closest to hand. (We have a shoe wardrobe – a fabulous double-sliding-door closet with the perfect height and depth shelves in our laundry. I know, so lucky!)

When I do all these things, I not only fall in love with my clothes all over again, but I feel the love being returned, as already mentioned briefly in Chapter 2. 'Fall in love with your current wardrobe'. I can actually sense the energy that my clothes and accessories feel appreciated and cherished. It's quite incredible really.

I am a spiritual person, but I am also very practical.

So for me to feel the loving energy emanating from my clothes, well, it blows my mind a little bit. And the best thing is that it feels really good. Just as you can catch a glow from someone who really, really likes you, so too will you feel the radiant warmth from your closet.

So that's the ethereal piece, and the practical piece is that you will save money without even meaning to. You will be so happy with your wardrobe and current clothing choices, that you won't want to go to the shops as much. Your clothing really will look far more appealing when looked after and neatly stored, just as a retail store makes their stock more attractive by displaying it neatly and nicely, as mentioned in the previous chapter.

Perhaps there might be a few gaps that you find when going into a new season, and you can go out specifically for those items, but apart from that you will probably feel content and serene.

And the nice thing is that when you do go for a browse, whether it's at the mall or online, your energy will be very different. Much calmer, and you won't have to hold onto yourself to avoid buying everything you see. Your shoulders will drop with a peaceful feeling, your breathing will become deeper and you will see shopping for what it is: a chance to find out what is new and beautiful, and be able to appreciate it without owning it, unless it is something that you really could see elevating your current clothing collection.

Most of the time I don't let my closet get so far out

of hand like when my husband ran out of underwear. Most of the time I do laundry regularly and keep on top of things. But you know when life just seems to be speeding away on you and you're in danger of being left behind? Yeah, those times. They happen.

That's when I notice the biggest difference in how I feel about my clothes – when I've had to do a marathon catch-up. I guess the silver lining is that I get to experience the immense feeling of wellbeing that comes from 'could try better' to 'top marks'. It is such a nice feeling!

But I am going to contribute to it intentionally from now on by keeping my wardrobe nice, and cultivating that 'in love' feeling – and getting the love back – from my lovingly tended closet.

Your Chic Closet Tips:

Next time you are doing your laundry and putting clothes away, **switch your mindset** from that of a chore begrudgingly done, **to one of positivity and appreciation**.

Appreciate your clothes, and the **items that belong to your family** too. It's almost easier when I am putting my husband's clothes away, because I can feel the loving care directed at *him*. I also appreciate that our clothes keep us warm (or cool), help us feel our best, and that we have so much to choose from. We really are all so lucky!

Chapter 10.
The two-colour rule

Years ago, I read a great interview with a French woman living here in New Zealand, and I was intrigued when she said that she 'always dresses by the two-colour rule'.

That one sentence in the article sent me on a hunt to find out more. Did she only wear two colours ever? Or in one outfit? What about prints? One of my all-time favourite combos to wear is denim and grey marle, with tan accessories, so I am torn. Is this three colours, or do accessories not count?

It was a fun research exercise. Of course I know I get to choose what I wear, but it's fascinating learning from a different perspective, and especially a French one, because we all know that French women have magical superpowers when it comes to style.

I decided to try it for myself and limit my outfits

to two colours. Because one of my main wardrobe staples is blue jeans, one of those two colours has to be navy, or grey-blue.

Even though I have some favourite three-colour combos (grey/denim/tan, grey/denim/black), I have to admit I did feel rather chic in my two-colour outfits. The phrase 'elegant restraint' came to mind.

I wore jeans with a navy V-neck fine cotton-knit top and beige high heels, with a beige trench-coat. Accessories-wise I wore a chunky gold necklace and a beige/tan/gold bag.

Another time I wore jeans, black heeled boots and a grey-blue V-neck cotton/silk jersey. You may notice a pattern forming. Actually my second example wasn't even two colours I've just realized. I also wore a classic Burberry-style print silk scarf. I'm a style rule rebel it seems.

My other wardrobe staples for everyday wear are white, off-white, grey, and black (slightly shiny) jeans, which gives me a break from having to choose blue as one of my two colours, phew!

I plucked up the courage to ask my French beauty therapist, Veronique, about the existence of this mysterious two-colour rule because, of course she'd know, being a French woman, right?

Do you want to know what she said? She *had never heard of it* and laughed a little tinkly laugh. She did know what the person being interviewed was getting at though. She said, 'People here, they are so...' and then threw her hands up in the air and shook them all around. Basically, we wear everything at once. I asked her how it was different in France. 'People are more... classy, classic'.

I felt a bit silly asking her, but I'm so glad I did. The curiosity would have burned me up otherwise.

I had the thought that the two-colour rule could apply to clothing items only, if I chose to employ it. Accessories which include scarves, belts and shoes are not included (within reason, of course).

When I think about my wardrobe (and also my dream wardrobe), I will mostly wear only two colours in my clothing, but maybe elevate it a little with different shoes or a scarf.

Perhaps for some of us, it might make things simpler and less cluttered in our clothing choices. It can get hard to match or coordinate more than two colours. Keep things simple and life is easier (or at least getting dressed is).

I've discovered that the two-colour rule suits me down to the ground, when I do it my way, which is two colours in my clothing with an accent colour in accessories, as already mentioned. Others may take a more flamboyant approach.

At least I don't have to be stricken with horror that I can no longer wear three colours because a French woman said so! But when you think about it, French women are very temperate, or at least the idealized ones are. They famously eat in moderation; and wear low-key items that compliment each other in subtle ways, rather than shop like a magpie and have a wardrobe full of things that have caught their eye.

I love to wear a lot of neutrals, and brighten things up with my scarf or shoes. I haven't bought a pair of black shoes in a long time, instead choosing tan, leopard, red, tangerine, hot pink and black/white snake print! They look crazy all together in my closet, but when I wear grey jeans and a white shirt, I feel so good in my hot pink tab-front loafers.

Another thing to consider is that the less colours you wear at the same time, the more expensive everything looks (which I expand upon in Chapter 4. 'Cultivating the expensive look). An outfit all in navy, or tones of oatmeal and winter-white can look luxurious and elegant to the eye.

But that's the fun of dressing yourself. One day you can be that mysterious lady in black, with big sunglasses on, and the next you'll go out in shades of spring pinks. It's nice to be able to use colour this way. Wear what you love to wear and be yourself; you don't need to impress anybody *but* yourself.

Your Chic Closet tips:

Try the two-colour rule just for fun. You might find new favourite ways to wear items that you already own. Then again, if you find it too restrictive, you'll know it's not for you.

What works for someone else might not be *your* thing, and that's a wonderful truth to remember in life. While this is a chapter about the two-colour rule, **the most important thing is that you embrace what you love**. If you love wearing twelve colours all at once, do it and feel great. I feel my best in simple, clean lines with not too much going on. It clears my head. But on the odd occasion when I feel like piling everything on, I do it, and I do it with pleasure and gusto.

Chapter 11.
Inspiring yourself to slim with your wardrobe

Have you ever found yourself sick of being cut in half by your jeans, muffin top spilling over? And of having panic attacks that you would not have anything to wear if you grew out of your largest size jeans? I have, and it's not much fun.

In a situation like this in the past, I had the epiphany to create a small capsule wardrobe in my current size. Not the size I wished I was, or could be with a crash diet, but being entirely realistic and figuring out what to do about dressing myself – and feeling good about it – exactly as I was.

I decided to create a capsule wardrobe of everything that fitted me, *including my nicest clothes*. Not an evening dress, obviously, nothing like that, but dressier clothes that I normally deemed 'too good' for everyday wear.

At the time, I had one pair of jeans and one pair of trousers that fitted me, so I started my collection with those. Then I went through all my tops and put aside the ones that pinched my upper arms or clung unforgivingly around the torso area. Piece by piece I went through my wardrobe and gathered everything that was comfortable and would flatter me.

This is the **first step: find everything that fits you well**.

I had blouses/shirts that I was usually too lazy to iron, but because I had changed my mindset from, 'Urgh, so much ironing', to, 'Create a capsule wardrobe to feel good in', I happily ironed them straight away so they were ready to wear. From this I had three more lovely choices and saw that I was doing **step two: have everything ready to go**.

I got out my pilling 'shaver' and whizzed over two tops that had a bit of rubbing, making them look like new again. I have neglected maintaining my clothes at times, as detailed in Chapter 9. 'The spiritual aspect to looking after your clothes', with washing and drying them being the only things I did. But when I gave myself the time to care for my clothes by ironing, de-pilling, doing minor repairs, cutting loose threads, and removing scratchy labels, everything looked more appealing and I had more choices.

I could see my new slim capsule coming together. It was such a thrill!

This little project of curating a slim capsule wardrobe helped me in more ways than just finding outfits to wear without going shopping.

- I started to appreciate what I had.

- The focus was taken off snacking and onto something more productive.

- I felt like I was taking care of my possessions and therefore myself.

- I received the satisfaction of curating my own capsule wardrobe and seeing how nice it looked in my closet.

- I was taken out of my head (where I indulged in too much over-analysis and focusing on my problems, which just made them worse) and into action which was far more calming.

- I no longer felt self-conscious in clothing that was too tight.

From putting together my capsule collection, I was quite surprised that I had a reasonable number of outfit options (even with just a few pairs of trousers) and it took the pressure off how I was feeling about my weight.

And because I felt less stressed with tight clothes no longer digging in and reminding me how much I'd been overindulging, it actually made it easier to eat better and resist the sweet treats I had been soothing myself with. It's crazy, because you think it would be the opposite – that tight clothing would make you not want fattening food. But what happens with me is I go the way of, 'I feel like crap and nothing fits, so I'm going to eat something yummy to feel better'. It's not logical, but it's where my mind went to.

I felt great about my 'new' capsule wardrobe and excited about getting dressed in the morning, which was a delightful change, I can tell you. I dug out my scarves and jewellery and was inspired to add the extra touches.

This good feeling (which is **step 3 – have fun getting dressed each day**) continued with me being inspired by clothing in general, inspired by looking and feeling good and it got me back into the mindset of caring how I looked and caring about being slim. When I was the other way, I cared on an intellectual level how I looked, but ahead of that I just cared about eating something delicious and decadent.

Separate the sizes

When you remove the smaller sizes from your closet you can see what is left and work with that, rather than be faced every single morning with the horribly demotivating question of, 'What can I fit?'

With my temporary capsule wardrobe, I decluttered very little. We do have a few consignment stores in New Zealand, but it's not as popular as in other countries, so when I get rid of things, they are donated or thrown out. This makes me more careful when buying, otherwise I have to literally give clothing – and money – away. For this reason too, I am more than happy to keep smaller-sized clothing in a different area. It doesn't worry me that it's there but it's certainly nice not to have to flick past those pieces every morning.

Getting more involved in creating my own personal style is when I tend to snack less, and curating a right-sized wardrobe helps kickstart this when I have temporarily lost my way. When I am researching Chanel (more in the next chapter!) or an elegant and classical way of dressing for example, nibbling junk foods seems less attractive. A crisp glass of Perrier or a steaming hot tea or coffee is much more civilized between meals. I'm sure Coco Chanel did not bolt down low-quality chocolate just because she was bored or felt flat that day.

What also belongs in my slim closet is self-love. I don't beat myself up if something doesn't look great on me. I either declutter it if it's the correct size but perhaps isn't a flattering shape or colour, or put it away if it's a little snug, feeling excited for when I am able to fit it again soon.

Life really is too short and precious to stress, and did you know that the stress hormone cortisol makes you put on weight? Just another reason to focus on fashion and your personal style instead of trying to avoid snacking.

Your Chic Closet Tip:

Keep this chapter in your back pocket, and use it if you find yourself in a similar, 'Help! I can't fit anything!' situation. I know you will find it just as useful as I did. And remember: **self-love. We have too little time on this earth to consider anything else**. Treat and talk to yourself like you would a dear friend – your best friend!

Chapter 12.
Fashion versus style
a la *Coco Chanel*

Whenever I spritz on a Chanel perfume or visit the Chanel website, I feel so stylish, chic and inspired. I then vow to myself that I am *only* going to wear Chanel fragrances, dress in black, cream and white (with navy and white stripes for casual) and have a home decorated in black, cream and burnt ochre with gilt touches.

Yes, I am prone to thoughts of extreme action.

I won't be doing any of this though, because I enjoy variety too much, but Mademoiselle Chanel's legacy does inspire me to live in a more elegant, thoughtful and creative way, which will help me not get drawn into the trashy side of things (such as reality television, low-quality foods and gossipy websites).

She is also an inspiration to stop looking around at what others are doing, and *do it for myself*. I highly doubt, if the Daily Mail website had been around when Coco was alive, that she would have read it each morning with her café crème. *Non*, Coco would have been starting her day deciding if she was going to ride her horse, meet a friend in her local café, or head straight to her atelier to create another design.

Rather than read about someone else who has started a successful business, she would go out and start her own successful business, such as her first boutique in Deauville. Yes, she was a person who made things happen.

I loved the book *Mademoiselle: Coco Chanel/Summer 62* (also published as *Coco Chanel: Three Weeks/1962*). It is entirely comprised of black-and-white photos, from when young American photographer Douglas Kirkland documented Coco during the creation of her summer 1962 fashion collection.

In the early pages she is photographed walking to work through the streets of Paris, paparazzi style. She looks like she could wear the same clothing today, and her hair, makeup, and pearls are classic and modern at the same time. It's only the people and vehicles around her that give the decade away.

I enjoy looking stylish and like I've made an effort, but I'm not so much into fashion. I'm more likely to be inspired by these old photos of

Mademoiselle Chanel than I am the latest Vogue.

One of my core values is 'simplicity', which I think Coco shared, and I love applying this to all aspects of my dress:

- *Simplicity of line (the cut) in my chosen clothing items*
- *Simplicity in colour palette*
- *Simplicity in my closet with not too many pieces*
- *Simplicity in that most of my pieces are a solid colour and a few stripes; only one or two items have a print*

Even with accessories I don't like to have too many. When my box of scarves was too much for me, I took a few out for the season and stored the rest.

The essence of Chanel

What inspires me most is my internal vision of signature Chanel at the time she was doing her thing. She truly was a visionary lady who impacted fashion and even the way we live, all these years later. To be as gutsy as she was now would be something, but back then? Outstanding.

I love to keep the spirit of Chanel in my mind so I can enjoy that feeling without having to dress exactly like her. I always feel inspired by her but it's a feeling rather than a way to look.

It's the same with other style icons. I admire Diane Keaton's unique style of dress which I wouldn't necessarily wear verbatim, but I can be inspired by her courage to dress in a way that most pleases her, and I think she always looks great.

The most important thing in creating your own style of chic, is deciding what you love first and building on that. I have always been drawn to the classics. You might be different, and have other influences you love to draw upon.

However, I think we can all agree that having inspiration to move us forward is useful, and I often invite my inner Chanel to help me make decisions when shopping, or dressing each morning.

My Chanel connection

To finish this chapter, would you allow me to share my personal Coco bond with you?

In 1969 my grand-aunt lived and worked as a nurse at the American Hospital in Paris, *and cared for Coco Chanel.* One evening Mademoiselle Chanel did not feel up to having a bath, so had my grand-aunt empty bottles of Chanel No. 5 into a basin for a sponge bath. When she was finished, my grand-aunt was instructed to pour the fragrance down the sink.

During the same hospital stay, a very young Karl Lagerfeld came in to see Coco, among other visitors.

When I asked my grand-aunt if Coco spoke much, she said she never *stopped* talking, however it was in very fast French and my grand-aunt was still learning to speak the language at that stage so didn't catch much at all. Such a shame! Imagine having a conversation with Coco Chanel and the questions you could ask her.

Your Chic Closet Tip:

Consider what your fashion/style ratio is. For me it's a high proportion of style with a smidge of fashion to liven things up. Yours might be a much higher percentage of fashion. I always admire those who constantly pop out with the latest thing, and it is appealing, but I have to be true to myself.

Contemplate what makes *you* most happy and honour that spirit in your closet.

Chapter 13.
How to be a frugal fashionista

I am a thrifty girl at heart and would always rather spend less, than more, when adding new items to my wardrobe. This is not a new thing for me. I remember in my late teens and early twenties one of my best-loved books was a Vogue publication with lots of inspiring eighties-tastic pictures called *More Dash Than Cash* by UK Vogue journalist Kate Hogg.

What I learned from this book and other sources such as magazine articles that I wished I'd torn out, is that it's not just about buying new things. It's how you style your clothes, accessorize, do your hair and makeup, and tweak your appearance to be fashionable while still honouring your classic and minimalist preferences. Hmm, sounds a lot like the idealistic French Chic style, doesn't it? Fascinating.

In this chapter, I want to share with you my favourite ways to be a frugal fashionista; to be inspired by fashion (even if you are a classics girl like me) and create your own stylish look without spending a lot of money.

First, you need to go through your closet before you even step foot in a store. I know this will probably sound boring when you are just itching to go shopping, but it's truly the only way you can get a handle on things. Familiarize yourself with what you have, especially if it's at the change of a season or even if it's not. Get everything out and expose your clothes to the light of day. When I did this I found I had seventy-five clothes hangers with items I loved on them. Seventy-five!

That told me I didn't need to go shopping just yet as I was in no danger of running out of clothes. Even if some of them were my bathrobe, special occasion and outerwear, there were certainly plenty of wearable everyday clothes.

Create a capsule wardrobe for right now. I go into more detail in Chapter 11. 'Inspiring yourself to slim with your wardrobe', but wanted to include a brief description in this chapter as well, because seeing what you already have is a big part of being a frugal fashionista.

Take every item out (in your current size, if you fluctuate like I do), and put them on the bed. See if there are new combos you can make from them. Note the colour palette that will naturally occur because you have chosen all these items in the past.

Hopefully you love the palette!

It is here that you might see where there are strategic pieces missing. For me, I had plenty of tops but needed some new bottoms to go with them. Last winter I remember I had no warm tops but plenty of jeans and trousers. By doing this exercise you will know what you need to shop for, if anything. You may find that you already have everything you need for a chic minimal wardrobe for the current season.

Now you get to create some excitement and make it seem like you have new things, by **updating what you have**. I started noticing a lot of cropped, unhemmed jeans (with shaggy frayed edges) when I was out running errands a while back, and started researching the new Levi's 505C cropped jeans with ripped legs. I really didn't need any more jeans because I had quite a few pairs, and they are nice Diesel ones, but they all had long legs. None of them were cropped.

My solution was to take a deep breath and cut the bottoms off my most ripped and distressed looking pair. *Et voila*, 'new' jeans that have updated my look and I love wearing them. No expenditure necessary.

Wear your better items. After I went through my closet and took everything out, I made a capsule collection of those pieces which fit me nicely as well as being appropriate for the current season. I saw that there were quite a few items – mainly tops and blouses – that I chose not to wear very often because they were a little dressier.

I still don't wear them around the house, but if we go out for coffee, or to the movies, why not wear a beautiful blush-peach sueded silk blouse or something dressier than my everyday gear? When else am I going to wear it? I enjoy the good feeling of dressing up slightly more; I am wearing what I have; and it feels like I have bought something new. Wins all round.

Declutter, one category at a time. This is how you find treasures in your closet; the items that you bought and didn't realize how much you love them and how much wear you get from them. It can be overwhelming to think of everything in your wardrobe, so start with something simple; say scarves, shoes or maybe costume jewellery.

With my scarves, I started wearing them more in Autumn which makes sense. I had stopped wearing any scarves, even lightweight ones because I just wasn't in the mood over summer. But ever since I began laying out my clothes to create an outfit before I get dressed (see Chapter 17. 'Lay out your clothes'), it is fun to create a whole look by adding a scarf.

I have all my scarves in a fabric storage box with a lid on. I tipped the whole lot out on my bed and chose my absolute favourites *du jour* and what I thought would compliment my winter wardrobe. I decluttered a few that I knew I'd never wear again, and stored others that I still liked but didn't want to wear just now.

As I went through my closet category-by-category, I became more and more enthused, and by the end I had a very inspiring and streamlined wardrobe to entice me each morning.

Revisit your favourite fashion inspiration. Remembering that book *More Dash Than Cash* from my younger days sparked something fresh and new inside.

I love to channel the nineties when I am looking for inspiration, but not because I want to wear matte makeup and block-heeled shoes (both of which I loved at the time, coveting the outfits on television series *Melrose Place*.) To me, the essence of the nineties says simplicity, minimalism, the sensual Calvin Klein aesthetic, and Carolyn Bessette-Kennedy's stunning style.

For you it may be your younger days love affair with Laura Ashley and the sprigged flower prairie dress. It's not that you want to go back in time and wear that exactly, but it helps you dream, and draw in your love of feminine fashion if you've temporarily forgotten about it.

Try looking in discount stores first. When I did identify that I needed more to wear on my lower half, I decided to start my shopping at less expensive stores. Spending a lot is not necessarily a guarantee of something being better quality or more flattering to your body shape. I have seen plenty of dreadfully cut clothing items on bargain racks that I wouldn't even pay $10 let alone $300 for. I like to think I have a healthy distrust of clothes that cost too much.

Yes, some items you can see the quality, but some don't look as much as the price on the tag at all. I like to start my shopping trips at the least expensive places first, just to see what's around. If I find what I am looking for at a great price, I stop there, and if not, I move up a notch.

I'm not advocating buying cheap clothes entirely, but don't avoid them altogether either. There can be some real gems to be found, and the quality can be okay too. I like to have a high-low mix in my closet, just like the fashionistas do. Mixing inexpensive with designer makes both look better, and your style budget goes further as well.

Your Chic Closet Tip:

Choose the point from this chapter that appeals the most, and put it into action. Browse an inexpensive store online for research; declutter one category; or go and look up your former favourite style inspiration – *Sex and the City*? *Melrose Place* like me? *Friends* even?

Chapter 14.
Creating the perfect wardrobe for you

What do you think of when you read 'the perfect wardrobe'? Would it be certain brands represented, total luxury, shoes on shelves up to the ceiling?

For me, the perfect wardrobe would be perfect pieces that make me look amazing, no matter my weight. There would be a moderate number of items, which all mix and match to make getting dressed a breeze. Everything suits my lifestyle and what I get dressed for each day, and it's easy-care too.

Denim forms the basis of my wardrobe, because I love it, so there would be plenty of that in my perfect wardrobe. I have denim jeans as well as light-weight denim dresses for when it's hot. Who says you can't wear denim year-round?

Having periodic clean-outs keeps my wardrobe feeling perfect too. I don't throw that much away; gone are the days of my closet being like a merry-go-round where I bought a lot and donated a lot. Now I take pleasure from buying only just enough and really appreciating what I have. When something is worn out or tired looking, it goes into the rag bin.

I think what is wonderful is that each of our closets will be completely different, but we can all cultivate a perfect closet; one that works for our lifestyle, and fits within our budget, and hopefully gives us pleasure instead of pain each day when we are getting dressed.

If there was one item I wouldn't be without, apart from jeans, it would be my small collection of **summer dresses**. Nothing is easier or cooler to wear when it's hot, and once you have found the shape that flatters you, you're golden. I usually buy two or three new dresses each year, and rotate them heavily throughout the hottest summer months.

I know for me that I can't have a horizontal waist seam (I am busty and short-waisted with long legs and it makes my body look even shorter), preferring a shift-type dress with vertical darts. Once I saw this, it went on my personal style guidelines list. Finishing just above the knee feels like a good length too, which I usually wear with flats, going into wedge sandals if I want to feel a bit special.

I have always been envious of those who have a clear vision of their personal (clothing) style and the appropriate edited wardrobe.

At any one time I will have a couple of different sizes of clothing and if not plentiful styles, more than one. Every time I think of having a huge cleanout I think, 'What if I lose weight? What if I change my mind?'

I am constantly thinking of ways I can streamline my wardrobe into its most perfect and purest form, and having guidelines that I have collected over time helps with this.

Identifying your 'perfect wardrobe'

When I think of my perfect wardrobe, I keep coming back to the French Chic style. It's a very broad generic term and really covers whatever someone wants to put under that genre. What I choose to put it under are true classics, cut to a flattering fit, and with a French touch in the colour palette and style. Pieces I have already which fit the bill are:

Flattering t-shirts in cotton with a tiny amount of elastane – in white, black and true red. They have a scoop neck to minimize my bust (not 'v' or crew) with short sleeves which flare out a little, so they don't cling and emphasise my upper arm.

Perfectly fitting jeans. Finding a perfectly fitting jean is a work in progress, and we all know there is a huge difference between styles. I have bought expensive jeans and cheaper jeans, and I have to say:

I've had more success with cheaper jeans! I know this goes against fashion advice ('always buy good jeans') but it's just how it has worked out for me lately. And I live in jeans, so I don't want to spend a lot of money and have them be worn out quickly from daily wear, or getting charcoal marks on them from lighting the wood burner at night.

Flattering and **slightly dressy sleeveless tops**. I have a couple that I wear when it's really hot in the summer. They drape over the shoulder so are more glamorous than a basic cotton tank top but are still cool to wear in the heat.

Beige cotton **knee-length trench coat**, which I love. I bought it in Paris on my first-and-only-so-far trip in 2001. Paris is a really, really long way from where I live. Until next time I make do and daydream. And wear my trench. I know the trench coat is such a French cliché, but what can I say? I love it!

I also have a short beige cotton trench-style coat bought from a très-inexpensive store. I unpicked the label, sewed in a few loose threads and haven't looked back. I wear it more than my long coat even though the long coat has a far better pedigree.

LBD. I know the little black dress is not for everyone, but I adore mine. I wore it to my cousin's wedding with red-and-white polka dot sling backs, and a white leather handbag which had a red-and-white polka dot silk scarf tied around the handle.

Along with classic clothing goes the classic accessories:

A **Cartier Tank Française** stainless-steel-and-gold small-size watch which I have worn every day for the past twenty years and will wear for the rest of my life. I bought it for myself for my thirtieth birthday as a newly single woman. It seemed a crazy purchase at the time, but it had been my dream watch for many years. Because of the dual-tone metal it can be worn with both gold and silver jewellery. I love a fabulous watch because not only is it a useful item, but it can double as a piece of jewellery as well.

A small wardrobe of earrings – real pearl studs, faux diamond studs and small-to-medium yellow gold hoops. I always, always wear earrings and love the lift they give to my look, even while at home in loungewear or casual daywear.

A few necklaces – my main ones are cultured baroque pearls or a chunky gold necklace with French coin attached. I always have the quandary of 'should I wear earrings and a necklace, and then how do I wear a scarf at the same time. My personal opinion of what I feel comfortable in is earrings and a scarf, or necklace and nothing else (but then I miss wearing earrings and a scarf!) If I wear a scarf around my neck, then I usually forego a necklace (but I have worn pearls with a scarf in the past). If I feel like I still need a scarf, I will tie it on my handbag.

The packing plan

Packing to go away on a trip is a great time to practise your 'perfect wardrobe'. When I travelled to my cousin's wedding I flew there, so I could only take only what I would definitely be wearing (as opposed to driving there, when you can pack everything you might ever need).

This necessitates a plan: what am I doing for each day and what should I wear, right down to accessories.

It's actually really fun, and for a staycation we had a while back at the Westin hotel, I even took photos of what I packed because I was enjoying myself so much. I love those magazine interviews where someone stylish shows their favourite things (they always include Diptyque candles, always!)

My Westin wardrobe was sort of like that, because it wasn't just the going-out clothes, but the lounge wear, what I was going to read, the perfume I was taking etc. It gave me a flavour for the night we were staying there.

Packing for a trip is definitely a fun way to create your perfect wardrobe, even if temporarily. Dreaming of that trip and seeing how nice it looks to only have the pieces which you consider to be your best and most appropriate for your wonderful holiday can kickstart the thoughts of, 'Well, why am I keeping all this other stuff then?'

Paring down your wardrobe is a constant process through the years. And it's fascinating to see how your style evolves and how much your taste changes. I try not to stay stuck in one style or mindset, even with my beloved idealistic French Chic style. I keep coming back to it, but I also remain open-minded and continually seek out new style icons to keep my look fresh and modern, while still being me.

Your Chic Closet Tips:

Consider **what outfits you wear the most** in each season, and start to build more looks around these when you need to replenish your wardrobe.

Ask yourself what your **absolute favourite looks** are and wear those more often.

If you have **a style that you keep going back to**, like my classic French style, just run with it. Sometimes I think I shouldn't do the French cliché thing, but if I truly love striped boat-neck tops with bracelet-length sleeves, what's the harm?

Peruse your Pinterest board for outfits, and see what is represented there. Does it resemble your own wardrobe? Why the disconnect? I've found it fun to **recreate a pinned outfit right down to the last detail**. I have been thrilled with the results, and found new ways to wear the clothes I already own.

Often those street style images have been carefully curated by seasoned stylists, so make good use of their expertise and **learn from the way they do things**!

Chapter 15.
Be inspired by men

I love to note what other women are wearing, whether it's in real life or at the movies, but I am often just as inspired by well-turned-out men. So much so that I have started a Pinterest board called 'Inspiring Men' (under my account 'fifileparisgirl'), to collect the images in one place.

It all started off with the James Bond movie 'Spectre', that I went along to with my husband. I write more about how this movie made me consider males as style role models in my book *Financially Chic*, but I want to say again here, Daniel Craig impressed me by the way he held himself, and with the clothes he wore in the movie.

He dressed *exquisitely*. He walked in a masterful way and owned the scenes he was in. He had ease, grace, elegance, and his own personal power. It was partly the character he played, and partly Daniel

Craig, the actor.

Of course, to be playing this role he needed to be in the leanest and healthiest shape he could possibly be, which made his clothes look fantastic. But it was more than just his physical beauty. He had a presence and a magnetism which made everything he wore almost crackle with electricity.

From experiencing this movie, I can put on my Daniel Craig cloak when I want to feel powerful and strong. And I can still do this in my own feminine way. I'm not going to stride around in a tuxedo jacket, but borrowing the vibe of his character helps me take that extra little bit of effort when getting ready for my day, not nibbling just because food is there, and making big plans for myself to inspire my actions.

Another male who inspires me is Jeff Goldblum. I don't know how he did it, but he went from quite a geeky guy who played quirky characters to a smartly dressed style icon with his signature chunky spectacles. His body moves languidly and in a driven way, all at the same time.

And he plays piano in a jazz bar in New York City. I mean come on, the man is seriously cool. I think I first noticed his metamorphosis through his character in the movie *Le Weekend*. Plus, *Le Weekend* is set in Paris, so bonus points.

My third male style icon is Mark Francis Vandelli. He first came onto my radar from watching the English reality show *Made in Chelsea*. *Made in Chelsea* is one of my guilty pleasures when I don't want to have to think too much. I love to be inspired by the young, rich, and beautiful people from London's Chelsea suburb.

Mark Francis is my favourite character in this show. He holds himself apart from the others slightly; he does not get involved in fighting or drama, and instead has his own stylish storyline asides, with witty Oscar Wilde-style quotes and a fun over-the-top snobbishness.

His Instagram page @markvandelli is filled with glamorous globe-trotting – mostly in Europe and the United Kingdom, with pithy captions and beautiful surroundings. He dresses in a very well-bred Euro-chic kind of way, and he too inspires me to keep my standards high and not worry too much about what others might think.

When I saw that an increasing number of my style icons were male, I tried to work out what that meant. I didn't desire to wear man tailoring or dress like Diane Keaton (although I love her style on her, alas my bust size means I would never be able to pull off her look).

What I think catches my eye in a sartorial way, is, as I have mentioned with my specifics above, their inner power. The way they carry themselves, have confidence in themselves and dress how they dress, without apology.

In New Zealand there is the tall poppy syndrome, where you could be (figuratively) cut down for rising too high and being too overly confident. Confidence was not an admirable trait when I was growing up!

So to see these men being so masterful and aligned with their own power, it's something I want to emulate the feminine version of. It means dressing how I would most love to and feeling good about that.

It's quite fascinating that something others might consider frivolous and shallow (such as putting the time into curating your wardrobe to best reflect your true self), actually turns out to be more of a psychology lesson.

And we can all remember those times when we had an outfit on that felt good and we were *invincible*. I went to sign some real estate paperwork with my husband yesterday, and I wore high heels and a spritz of 'power' perfume. These two things changed skinny jeans and a linen tunic shirt into me feeling like a boss when I walked into that property broker's office!

I love that with your clothing you can feel bullet proof when going out into the world, and cozy, cosseted and safe while relaxing at home. All by using different pieces of fabric stitched in different ways. It's amazing when you think about it!

So, take notice of who you are inspired by, and don't dismiss them just because they are a different sex to you, live in a different culture or country, or have a different lifestyle to you.

Your Chic Closet Tips:

When you are drawn to someone, pick apart just why.

Is it their softness?
Their strength?
The colours they wear?
The fact that they show their minimalist closet?
They look like they're having fun with their wardrobe?
Everything is thrifted?

Just what appeals? Dig down and write out everything you can think off, then look back at your findings.

For me with my inspiring men, I take away that I want to add more of these things into my everyday dress:

- Tailored blazers to top off an outfit – I have them, but don't often wear them

- High heels that are both powerful and comfortable (I'm sure they are out there somewhere)

- Taking pride in my appearance and feeling good

about myself

- Dressing to impress me, before trying to impress anybody else

You can see on my list that it is both what I wear and how I wear it. You may well find it is the same for you, so take a look at your fashion inspirations and have fun with this!

Chapter 16.
The chic lingerie drawer

Over the past years I have upgraded my lingerie and continue to do so once or twice a year or when I see that it is necessary. I did it again recently and enjoyed buying a few new pieces.

Even though I might like pieces when I am out browsing, I sometimes pass them by. This might be if they are pretty but a bit mumsy (I am drawn to that look!) or practical and comfortable but with not enough elegance (I want everything in the one package).

My desire with lingerie is to have it be 'sexy and sophisticated'. These are the two words I keep in mind when I am out shopping or deciding what to keep when I am going through my lingerie drawer. I elaborate on this concept in 'Day 12. Curate your wardrobe like it is your own bijou boutique' in my book *Thirty Chic Days*.

I don't buy expensive underwear and I usually shop in sales. My most recent shopping trip I went to the 'nothing over $20' sale at a local outlet store. I spent $150, which is a lot for me, but I found three nice bras and several pairs of knickers. Also, a pair of satin drawstring trousers for home loungewear.

I am more adventurous with my lingerie these days and like to buy pretty colours and always in lace. I buy matching and semi-matching knickers to the bras and pair them up when I am dressing.

For example, if I have a black bra and black knickers, that's fine with me. They don't have to be from the same range. I have a grey lace bra with pink satin straps. I do have the matching knickers, but I also like to wear that bra with my pink lace knickers.

It has taken me some time to put the comfortable and utilitarian underwear mindset behind me. I still do have comfy knickers that I wear with my exercise gear to go for a walk, plus my sports bra of course; but when I get dressed after my shower I wear my lovely lacy lingerie, which hasn't always been the case in the past.

What I have taken from the idealistic French lady, is that underwear does not have to be entirely invisible. I don't mean to have all your lingerie hanging out and looking tacky, but if you can see a little bit of lace pattern through a top, or a peek of a coloured satin bra strap with a boat-neck top, that's okay with me.

I would far rather have the bright-coloured strap showing than a beige knit strap. Do you know what men think of smooth beige underwear? Not a lot. It is the biggest passion killer! My husband actually shuddered when I asked him what he thought of it. When he first mentioned this ages ago, I got rid of my beige smooth tee-shirt bra. It was near the end anyway, so it was a good time to upgrade to something more appealing.

And it makes me so happy to open my lingerie drawer these days. I have two KonMari-folded rows of lacy, colourful knickers and one row of older/comfy knickers for exercise, plus a small drawer of pretty bras.

When I find that my underwear selection feels a bit tired and things are looking shabby, it's time to have a go-through. Sometimes I don't need to go shopping if I get rid of some knickers and a bra, perhaps, because my selection suddenly looks much better with those few things gone. I never find myself too low on items because I usually come across a good sale before that happens.

There is nothing wrong with spending a lot of money on fancy lingerie if that's what you like, but for me, I am happy with mid-priced underwear. I wash it in the washing machine (with the bras in lingerie bags) and it comes out fine.

Embrace your femininity

Let's get pretty! We are feminine beings! Buy the colours you are drawn to and work out how to wear them with your clothes. Instead of that beige smooth bra under your white tee-shirt, why not a lace bra in soft peach or blush pink? There is not much difference between beige and blush, but *a world of difference* at the same time.

Even if you don't buy anything new right now, why not reorganize your lingerie drawer at least. Tip everything out on your bed and put it all back in neat folded rows, checking as you go if anything really does need to be thrown out. This instant mini-refresh will feel good and it will be so nice when you come to get dressed tomorrow morning. This is something you can do straight away without spending any money.

Look at your favourite pieces too – the ones you reach for most. What is your favourite type/colour/style etc? I don't like g's so much anymore, preferring the boy-leg, Brazilian, low-rise kind of brief. I like my bras lacy with underwire, and no padding.

Finding out these things about your preferred styles makes it easier when it is time to do a stock-up.

I hope this chapter has inspired you to take a fresh look at your lingerie style, because that is exactly how I shook things up for myself. One day, I looked at my underwear selection and saw what someone else might see – boring, tired, and unsupportive options in unexciting colours. I knew it was time to upgrade this area in my life.

Starting with the few things I needed and

choosing items that my stylish Parisian muse might when I needed more, meant I was stepping into the elegant bombshell I knew I was on the inside!

Your Chic Closet Tips:

First of all, **reorganize your underwear drawer**, and while you are doing this, cast a critical eye over everything. What do your pieces say about you? About how you take care of yourself?

Throw out the worst items, and if you don't have much left, **replace as you can** with comfortable, stylish options which suit your desired personal style. It might be 'sexy and sophisticated' like me, or 'playful and vibrant', 'soft and natural' etc. Just as you intentionally choose your clothes, so too is your intimate wardrobe an important part of your personal style, even if it is only you, and your husband, who sees it.

Enjoy feeling good in sensual underwear in black lace, plum, cinnamon or navy, or lighter shades such as peony pink, coral-red or fresh white; even if you are not the thinnest thing in the world (I'm certainly not). No matter your size or shape, treat yourself to beautiful lingerie. There are so many beautiful colours around, and at every price point too. Some of my favourites have come from Victoria's Secret, and even Kmart!

Chapter 17.
Lay out your clothes

I have saved my favourite tip for reinvigorating the passion for your wardrobe until last. It is the most simple and well-known advice ever, but until you actually do it you won't see the power of it.

I have heard of people laying out their clothes for the next day since I was young. It seemed to me that it was quite a 'mature' (as in 'old lady') thing to do and I didn't really see what difference it could make. Surely if all your clothes were clean and hanging in your closet, you could just get dressed from there and save time?

It seemed like a pointless step to me and so I ignored the advice for years, decades even. Then, one day, I must have seen something that inspired me try it. It was probably Diane in Denmark on YouTube. She uses the Flylady system and talks about preparing an outfit the night before. I love her fun and light-hearted way of doing things, so if anyone could enthuse me about trying a new organizing trick it would be her.

What I found, is that it seems there is something magical that happens when you lay your clothes out. Perhaps it is having that extra step in between stepping out of the shower and getting dressed that lets you look at what you are going to wear through a different lens.

I know for me it lets me be more creative. I am less lazy with my choices. And I go the extra mile with my accessories.

When I get dressed as I go, putting on my jeans then deciding what top will go with it, I don't have a bird's eye, or stylist's, view. I only see what I look like by looking down. But when I hold items up and compare the colour of denim along my selection of tops to see what looks best, I choose differently - better.

I hang my two pieces together and see how well they complement each other. And I also take this time to quickly check the next day's weather on my phone to see if I need to go slightly warmer or slightly cooler. I then choose underwear that will suit the garment styles and colours and tuck these through the hangers as well. Next are shoes that suit, and socks if it is winter. Finally, I look at costume jewellery and/or a scarf that would top off my outfit. I always wear my watch, wedding ring set and a pair of stud or hoop earrings, but perhaps a chunky necklace or scarf would make my outfit pop.

All of this doesn't take very long, and it's a lovely way to wind down before bed. I notice that I have gratitude for all the choices available to me in my closet. And I also notice when something is looking a little tired and either needs some action with my lint shaver or to be donated, or cut up for rags. I have the time to do what is necessary.

When I have done all this, I feel peaceful and ready for a good night's sleep. It's a wonderful feeling.

Let's compare this to how getting dressed goes when you haven't laid your clothes out (going from my own experience). You go to your closet and look to see what you feel like wearing. It seems warm today, so you choose a light-weight top (later realizing you were still warm from your shower and a few hours later feel a little chilly). You wore the same thing only recently, but can't be bothered looking any further, so put it on and then choose a pair of jeans. Your underwear doesn't match, but that's okay, no-one knows but you. Next, shoes, and you're done.

It's just a nicer experience to lay your clothes out, or at least it is for me!

And if you forget or are too tired to lay your clothes out at night, all is not lost. One day I simply forgot, so laid them out the next morning when I got up, before having my shower. It was just as effective as doing it the night before. So perhaps, depending on your schedule and whether you are a night or a morning person, you could choose to lay them out in the morning.

To recap, I resisted laying my clothes out for many years, then tried it. It worked well, and now I am a convert. However, that *still* doesn't mean I do it every day. The main reasons are that I am a little bit rebellious and also a little bit lazy; but the more I do it, the happier I feel. I can't help but think there must be something to that!

Your Chic Closet Tips:

There are a few different ways you can lay out your clothes, so don't worry if you are not the proud owner of a walk-in closet.

Some people have **a hook on the outside of their closet door**, for the purpose of hanging their next days' clothes on a hanger.

Or you could do what I did in our last home, and that is to **hang your outfit at one end of your clothes rail**.

Where I live now, we have a small walk-in closet with **hooks on one wall, so I hang my selection** there (doing this is also an incentive to keep those hooks clear).

And lastly, if you only choose your outfit on the day, make your bed before having your shower, and **lay the clothes out at the foot of the bed**. Doing this makes such a pleasing view when you come back into your bedroom, that it sets you up for a successful day!

21 top tips for a chic closet

To finish this book off, I'd love to share with you my top tips for a wardrobe that makes your stylish heart sing with joy.

I have thoroughly enjoyed writing *The Chic Closet*, and I hope you have gained loads of good ideas from reading it.

Remember, when it comes to getting dressed, it's all about *you, wonderful you*!

1. **Don't let the fear of making mistakes** or looking silly stop you from trying something new. If you see an outfit you'd like to try, who not do it? It doesn't need to be a drastic change from your normal look, but then again you might just decide to make a splash. Clothing, hair and makeup are all temporary and interchangeable, so if you're in the mood for something different, go for it!

2. **Notice what others are wearing**. People-watch and take in new ideas. It could be a colour combination that stands out (in a good way) on someone with a similar complexion to you.

I am also inspired to uplevel my way of dressing when I see someone who has really made an effort. In turn this helps me choose something out of the ordinary from my own wardrobe and to be that person for others.

Whenever I see someone stylish, with clothing on that I think I would like to wear, if possible I compliment them on their look and ask them where they got a particular item from. So far people have been happy to tell me. I do this is a conversational way, not in a 'whip out my clipboard' way.

3. **Be pressed, be chic**. One of my most slender, stylish and elegant friends went on a Scandinavian cruise a few years back, and told me that she asked for an iron to be brought to her cabin because she irons everything, absolutely everything she wears - she just cannot *not* iron her clothes.

I found that really cute, and if her love of ironing is how she always looks so polished, I'll take it.

4. **Stay ready**. Imagine how easy it would be to look great every day with minimal effort if

everything in your closet was clean, pressed, in good condition, fitted you well and was basically ready to wear. Imagine if you had clean hair in a good style for your hair type, a simple and pretty makeup routine ready to go, and smooth, moisturized skin. Imagine if you were happy with your body and fitted everything you owned.

It would be so straightforward getting dressed in the morning, and likely a lot of fun too. No mental anguish! That's the idea behind the 'Stay ready' phrase; 'When you stay ready, you don't need to get ready'.

It has been a game changer for me and something I am continually working towards because there are immense benefits.

5. **Dress up every day**. Start with the little things – wear earrings if you don't usually; lipstick and perfume too. Wear your dressier clothes occasionally. If it is hard to start dressing for your dream life, begin with baby steps. Just taking one little step can spark off all sorts of other things.

Something that has really helped me is to do the one thing that excites you and start with that, not what you 'think you should do'. Even if your thought is, 'It's late in the day, I'll do it tomorrow', all is not lost. Do it now! You will feel so good about yourself if you take a moment to brighten yourself up.

I promise because I do it too! I might touch up my makeup, brush and re-do my hair (if's up in a ponytail or chignon), put on some perfume and make sure I have a pair of earrings on.

6. **Channel your own inspiration.** Pretend you are the chic and elegant lady of your dreams and make it fun. Incredibly the 'pretend you' influences your real life in a good way – yay for that!

7. **Create a glow for your face.** I used to wear a lot of black but wear more colour now – I love red and other bright/feminine colours – all shades of blue, soft greens, buttermilk yellow... paired with white in the summer, or denim in the winter.

   And sparkle and shine too – think pearls or pretty necklaces. I like to make sure that whatever clothes, scarves, or jewellery are worn near my face add to and brighten up my face, rather than detract from it.

8. **Project self-confidence**, whether you have to fake it or not. Trick yourself into feeling good by owning the space you are in. Create your own confident vibe by standing taller, breathing in serenity and knowing that you are enough.

Other people can sense confident energy, and it's available to all of us.

9. **Shop with a high bar.** I have gotten pickier about fit and cut over the years – if a garment is not quite right, it goes back on the rack no matter how much I like it. An article of clothing is not going to change shape once I get home. It is hard to leave something, I know. But it is harder to live with clothes that don't fit you quite right. Hold out for only the absolute *Yesses* and over time you will build a wardrobe you love.

10. Want to **make your clothes instantly look better**, *and* look like you've lost five pounds? All you need to do is stand up straighter and pull your shoulders back and down. My favourite 'better in an instant' trick is to imagine a fine silk thread pulling me up from the crown of my head. It's incredible, but doing this helps me feel lighter and taller. (And it works whether you are standing up or sitting down – try it now!)

11. And another non-clothing personal style tip: **smile**. Smiling lifts all the muscles in your face which acts as a mini-facelift. You will instantly improve your looks, and feel happier at the same time.

12. If big department stores or shopping outlets overwhelm you, **stick to smaller stores**. I always have more luck when there are less options. And, knowing what I am looking for before I step foot into a store is a huge help too. So, I might be able to navigate a department store if I know I want a crisp white shirt. I can quickly scan areas while I walk around. And even before then, if you're in the mood, check out stores websites before you go shopping, just to do some research and see what is around.

13. **Style your closet** in a way that most pleases you: Buy inexpensive velvet and wooden hangers to give that boutique-style look; colour block your clothing; add a decorative hook to hang up the next day's outfit; have a small laundry hamper under your clothes to throw dirty clothes into if your laundry isn't near (our laundry is close, but I like to have that little hamper to hand, and I empty it every day or two into the bigger hamper in the laundry); hang stylish framed images if you have the wall space, or quotes and sayings that inspire you; fragrance your closet with sachets filled with fresh lavender, or keep a room spray or perfume in there and spritz it around every once in a while.

    The general idea is to make your closet a lovely place to visit!

14. **Give gratitude** for your clothes when they feel stale to you. This is an excellent pre-step to going shopping. So often when I do this, I regain appreciation for everything I own, and I am inspired to put together new outfits. It almost feels like I *have* been shopping, but I have not spent a cent.

15. **Go in with a colour scheme for the day**. I was in a feminine mood when dressing this morning. I still dressed in dark-wash jeans, which aren't a particularly feminine item of clothing, however, I chose a light mauve cashmere sweater, and tied a grape-purple gauzy silk scarf around my neck. To compliment this combo, I wore patent plum-coloured ballet flats.

    I felt really good about myself and it was a practical and easy-to-wear outfit, but I also honoured my feminine side too.

16. **Start your own personal style journal** where you note down styles that look particularly good on you, colours you love, colour combos you want to try, and all those sorts of yummy things. Include magazine pages where you love the outfit, and basically curate a place to arouse your personal style inspiration.

    I do have Pinterest boards like this, but I also

love my pen and paper version. It's a permanent, tangible source of stylish fun for me, and just opening it sets my heart aflutter!

17. What you loved in the past, style-wise, will probably still inspire you now. Your style will have evolved and you will likely wear current clothes, but if you look back at your favourite outfits then, you will probably find you are wearing today's version of the same thing. That's why it is a good idea, if you are feeling in a style rut (which I do from time to time), to **think back to your favourite looks** from the past. You will become re-excited about dressing yourself in a stylish way again. It sounds topsy-turvy, but it always works for me!

18. **Wear fabrics that feel pleasing to your skin**. Sometimes I wouldn't wear clothing items simply because I didn't want to, and when I asked myself, 'Why are you bypassing this pretty top, Fiona', it was because the fabric felt bad against my skin. I now know to avoid slithery knits (they feel as awful as they sound) and anything scratchy such as linen that is too rough. Having displeasing fabric touch my skin makes me grumpy! It just feels nicer and puts me in a better mood when I have nothing irritating my skin, so I am mindful of this now while out shopping.

19. You will have heard the helpful advice, 'Don't buy it just because it's on sale' which I agree with to a point, but I would also add, '**Don't be too suspicious of discounted items**'. I think you can build an incredibly stylish wardrobe shopping exclusively in sales. I love to grab a bargain, plus I am incredibly choosy about what I buy. Some of my favourite and most worn pieces have come from sales racks or special offers. The key is to be just as thoughtful about your purchase whether it is reduced in price or not.

20. **Round up all the 'It'll dos'** from your closet and put them on probation. I like to put all these items in a different area and, as I wear (and enjoy) them, put them back into my normal area once they have been washed. But if I didn't like wearing them, or keep finding reasons not to wear them, they are probably better off in the donation box.

    Or, to approach a similar thing from another angle, hang probation items on your closet rail at the far left or far right with something acting as a divider from your normal clothes (perhaps a hanger with a shopping bag over it like a suit cover?) As you wear clothes, once they are washed and returned to your closet, put them on the other side of the divider. As time goes by you will see what keeps getting passed over. Some say to force yourself to wear everything at least, and then it's easy to see what you need to clean out!

21. **Honour you. Be you, with all your heart.** Yes, it is nice to receive compliments from others, but ultimately the person who must be most happy with how you look is you. Dress in what makes you feel best. Have fun with your choices. Be physically comfortable. Wearing what you want to wear is just one of the many ways in which you can add to your happiness every single day. And when you feel amazing in what you are wearing, it shines out to others.

I love to see people dressed well, no matter their favoured personal style, age or size. And don't worry about standing out too much. It's far better than being invisible. Let's all put a little more passion into the way we dress and watch how the world brightens up! Enjoy!

A note from the author

Thank you so much for joining me in this fun personal style exploration. I think we can all elevate our look, and happiness, by experimenting with the way in which we dress ourselves. I love that in France, dressing well is considered to be a social service, because it is not just for you, it's for everyone who has to see you. Isn't that fabulous? I remember this when I am tempted to be a touch lazy, and it perks me right up.

And, when you know you look good, you feel good, which has a far-reaching effect on others because you are a happier, and nicer, person to be around. There is no downside to putting just a little more time and attention into your personal style.

If you enjoyed 'The Chic Closet', I would *so* appreciate an honest review on Amazon. It doesn't need to be long; just a few words would mean the world to me. Reviews, both good and bad, are so important to authors; it is how other people find their books. So, if you are happy to spend a few minutes writing a review, I thank you.

Have fun dressing yourself tomorrow!

See you soon,

Fiona

About the author

Fiona Ferris is passionate about and has studied the topic of living well for more than twenty years, in particular that a simple and beautiful life can be achieved without spending a lot of money.

Fiona finds inspiration from all over the place including Paris and France, the countryside, big cities, fancy hotels, music, beautiful scents, magazines, books, all those fabulous blogs out there, people, pets, nature, other countries and cultures; really, everywhere she looks.

Fiona lives in the beautiful and sunny wine region of Hawke's Bay, New Zealand, with her husband, Paul, their rescue cats Jessica and Nina and rescue dogs Daphne and Chloe.

To learn more about Fiona, you can connect with her at:

howtobechic.com
fionaferris.com
facebook.com/fionaferrisauthor
twitter.com/fiona_ferris
instagram.com/fionaferrisnz
youtube.com/fionaferris

Book Bonuses

http://bit.ly/ThirtyChicDaysBookBonuses

Type in the link above to receive your free special bonuses.

'21 ways to be chic' is a fun list of chic living reminders, with an MP3 recording to accompany it so you can listen on the go as well.

Excerpts from all of Fiona's books in PDF format.

You will also **receive a subscription** to Fiona's blog '*How to be Chic*', for regular inspiration on living a simple, beautiful and successful life.

Printed in Great Britain
by Amazon